MYOCARDIAL PROTECTION AND THE K_{ATP} CHANNEL

DEVELOPMENTS IN CARDIOVASCULAR MEDICINE

121. S. Sideman, R. Beyar and A. G. Kleber (eds.): Cardiac Electrophysiology, Circulation, and Transport. Proceedings of the 7th Henry Goldberg Workshop (Berne, Switzerland, 1990). 1991. ISBN 0-7923-1145-0.
122. D. M. Bers: Excitation-Contraction Coupling and Cardiac Contractile Force. 1991. ISBN 0-7923-1186-8.
123. A.-M. Salmasi and A. N. Nicolaides (eds.): Occult Atherosclerotic Disease. Diagnosis, Assessmentand Management. 1991. ISBN 0-7923-1188-4.
124. J. A. E. Spaan: Coronary Blood Flow. Mechanics, Distribution, and Control. 1991. ISBN 0-7923-1210-4.
125. R. W. Stout (ed.): Diabetes and Atherosclerosis. 1991. ISBN 0-7923-1310-0.
126. A. G. Herman (ed.): Antithrombotics. Pathophysiological Rationale for Pharmacological Interventions. 1991. ISBN 0-7923-1413-1.
127. N. H. J. Pijls: Maximal Myocardial Perfusion as a Measure of the Functional Significance of Coronary Arteriogram. From a Pathoanatomic to a Pathophysiologic Interpretation of the Coronary Arteriogram. 1991. ISBN 0-7923-1430-1.
128. J. H. C. Reiber and E. E. v. d. Wall (eds.): Cardiovascular Nuclear Medicine and MRI. Quantitation and Clinical Applications. 1992. ISBN 0-7923-1467-0.
129. E. Andries, P. Brugada and R. Stroobrandt (eds.): How to Face "the Faces" of Cardiac Pacing. 1992. ISBN 0-7923-1528-6.
130. M. Nagano, S. Mochizuki and N. S. Dhalla (eds.): Cardiovascular Disease in Diabetes. 1992. ISBN 0-7923-1554-5.
131. P. W. Serruys, B. H. Strauss and S. B. King III (eds.): Restenosis after Intervention with New Mechanical Devices. 1992. ISBN 0-7923-1555-3.
132. P. J. Walter (ed.): Quality of Life after Open Heart Surgery. 1992. ISBN 0-7923-1580-4.
133. E. E. van der Wall, H. Sochor, A. Righetti and M. G. Niemeyer (eds.): What is new in Cardiac Imaging? SPECT, PET and MRI. 1992. ISBN 0-7923-1615-0.
134. P. Hanrath, R. Uebis and W. Krebs (eds.); Cardiovascular Imaging by Ultrasound. 1992. ISBN 0-7923-1755-6.
135. F. H. Messerli (ed.): Cardiovascular Disease in the Elderly, 3rd ed. 1992. ISBN 0-7923-1859-5.
136. J. Hess and G. R. Sutherland (eds.); Congenital Heart Disease in Adolescents and Adults. 1992. ISBN 0-7923-1862-5.
137. J. H. C. Reiber and P. W. Serruys (eds.): Advances in Quantitative Coronary Arteriography. 1993. ISBN 0-7923-1863-3.
138. A.-M. Salmasi and A. S. Iskandrian (eds.): Cardiac Output and Regional Flow in Health and Disease. 1993. ISBN 0-7923-1911-7.
139. J. H. Kingma, N. M. van Hemel and K. I. Lie (eds.): Atrial Fibrillation, a Treatable Disease? 1992. ISBN 0-7923-2008-5.
140. B. Ostadal, N. S. Dhalla (eds.): Heart Function in Health and Disease. 1993. ISBN 0-7923-2052-2.
141. D. Noble and Y.E. Earm (eds.): *Ionic Channels and Effect of Taurine on the Heart.* Proceedings of an International Symposium (Seoul, Korea, 1992). 1993. ISBN 0-7923-2199-5.
142. H.M. Piper and C.J. Preusse (eds.): *Ischemia-reperfusion in Cardiac Surgery.* 1993. ISBN 0-7923-2241-X.
143. J. Roelandt, E.J. Gussenhoven and N. Bom (eds.): *Intravascular Ultrasound.* 1993. ISBN 0-7923-2301-7.
144. M.E. Safar and M.F. O'Rourke (eds.): *The Arterial System in Hypertension.* 1993. ISBN 0-7923-2343-2.
145. P. W. Serruys, D.P. Foley and P.J. de Feyter (eds.): *Quantitative Coronary Angiography in Clinical Practice.* 1993. ISBN 0-7923-2368-8.
146. J. Candell-Riera and D. Ortega-Alcalde (eds.): *Nuclear Cardiology in Everyday Practice.* 1993. ISBN 0-7923-2374-2.
147. P. Cummins (ed.): *Growth Factors and the Cardiovascular System.* 1993. ISBN 7923-2401-3.
148. K. Przyklenk, R.A. Kloner and D.M. Yellon (eds.): *Ischemic Preconditioning: The Concept of Endogenous Cardioprotection.* 1993. ISBN 0-7923-2410-2.

MYOCARDIAL PROTECTION AND THE K_{ATP} CHANNEL

Editors

Derek M. Yellon, Ph.D., DSc. MRCP(Hon), FESC, FACC

Professor of Cellular Cardiology
Head of the Division of Cardiology &
Director of the Hatter Institute
University College London Medical School & Hospitals,
London, United Kingdom

Garrett J. Gross, B.S., M.S., Ph.D.

Professor of Pharmacology & Toxicology
Department of Pharmacology & Toxicology
Medical College of Wisconsin
8701 Watertown Plank Road
Milwaukee 53226, USA

KLUWER ACADEMIC PUBLISHERS

Boston Dordrecht London

Distributors for North America:
Kluwer Academic Publishers
101 Philip Drive
Assinippi Park
Norwell, Massachusetts 02061 USA

Distributors for all other countries:
Kluwer Academic Publishers Group
Distribution Centre
Post Office Box 322
3300 AH Dordrecht, THE NETHERLANDS

Library of Congress Cataloging-in-Publication Data

Myocardial protection and the KATP channel / editors, Derek M.Yellon, Garrett J. Gross.
p. cm. -- (Developments in cardiovascular medicine : 179)
Includes index.
On t.p. "ATP" is subscript.
ISBN 0-7923-3791-3 (alk. paper)
1. Coronary heart disease--Chemotherapy--Congresses. 2. Calcium channels--Congresses. 3. Cardiovascular agents--Congresses.
I. Yellon, Derek M. II. Gross, Garrett J. III. Series.
[DNLM: 1. Myocardial Ischemia--metabolism--congresses.
2. Potassium Channels--metabolism--congresses. W1 DE997VME v. 179 1995 / WG 300 M99767 1995]
RC685.C6M976 1995
616.1'23--dc20
DNLM/DLC
for Library of Congress

Printed on acid-free paper.

Printed in the United States of America

Table of Contents

Contributing Authors

Professor Nicholas B Standen MA, PhD.
Professor of Physiology and Director
Ion Channel Group
Department of Cell Physiology & Pharmacology
University of Leicester
P.O.Box 138
University Road
Leicester LE1 9HN
United Kingdom

Professor Ulrich Quast PhD.
Head of Molecular Pharmacology Section
Department of Pharmacology
Section of Molecular Pharmacology
Medical Faculty
University of Tubingen
Wilhelmstr 56
D-72074 Tubingen
Germany

Mr Stefan Glocker
Department of Pharmacology
Section of Molecular Pharmacology
Medical Faculty
University of Tubingen
Wilhelmstr 56
D-72074 Tubingen
Germany

Professor David J Hearse Bsc, PhD, DSc, FACC.
Professor of Cardiuac Biochemistry and
Director of the Cardiovascular Research Unit
The Rayne Institute
St Thomas' hospital
London SE1 7EH,
United Kingdom

Dr Garrett J Gross BS, MS, PhD.
Professor of Pharmacology & Toxicology
Department of Pharmacology & Toxicology
Medical College of Wisconsin
8701 Watertown Plank Road
Milwaukee 53226
USA

Professor Derek M Yellon PhD, Dsc, MRCP(Hon), FESC, FACC.
Professor of Cellular Cardiology
Head of the Division of Cardiology &
Director of the Hatter Institute
University College London Medical School & Hospitals,
Grafton Way
London, WC1E 6DB
United Kingdom.

Professor Dr. Michiel .J Janse MD, PhD.
Professor of Experimental Cardiology
Department of Clinical and Experimental Cardiology,
M-0-052 Academic Medical Center
University of Amsterdam
Meibergdreef 9
1105 AZ Amsterdam ZO
The Netheralnds

Dr Authur M Wilde MD, PhD.
Consultant Cardiologist
Department. of Clinical and Experimental Cardiology,
M-0-0-52 Academic Medical Center
University of Amsterdam
Meibergdreef 9
1105 AZ Amsterdam ZO
The Netheralnds

Dr Henry J Purcell MB Bch, PhD.
Senior Research Fellow
The Royal Brompton Hospital
Sidney Street
London SW3 6NP
United Kingdom

Dr Kim M Fox MD, FRCP, FESC.
Consultant Cardiologist
The Royal Brompton Hospital
Sidney Street
London SW3 6NP
United Kingdom

Professor Lionel H Opie MD D Phil, FRCP.
Professor of Medicine and
Director of the Medical Research Council Ischaemic
Heart Disease Research Unit
University of Cape Town
Medical School
Observatory 7925
Cape Town
South Africa

Dr Gary J. Grover BS, MS, PhD.
Senior Principal Scientist
Department of Pharmacology
Bristol-Myers Squibb Pharmaceutical Research Institute
Route 206 & Provinceline Road
Princeton, N.J. 08543-400
USA

Preface & Acknowledgements

With the continual interest in developing means of protecting the ischemic and reperfused myocardium, as well as the advent of a particular excitement in the role that the K_{ATP} channel may play in this protection, we the editors, felt that it was both timely and appropriate that a concise, state of the art book, addressing this topic should be written.

A number of the concepts discussed in the following chapters were convened at a round table meeting held at Cliveden, England in 1995 under the auspices of the Cellular Biology Working Group of the European Society of Cardiology. We are grateful to Rhone Poulenc Rorer and Merck Lipha for providing an educational grant to sponsor the round table meeting and to support the publication of this book.

We also sincerely thank the Department of Academic & Clinical Cardiology at University College London and the Department of Pharmacology and Toxicology at the Medical College of Wisconsin for providing the academic environment that has enabled us to pursue our research and educational endeavours. On a more personnel note both Derek & Garrett particularly want to express their grateful thanks to Luci and Carol for their continued patience and understanding of our sometimes misguided drive to pursue our indulgence for academic gratification!

Finally our most sincere thanks must go to our distinguished contributors who despite the enormous pressures which are continually placed upon them all made contributions of the highest calibre. All the authors felt that a book addressing this important and highly topical subject should proceed without delay which we are delighted to say has allowed this volume to be published within one year of its conception.

Derek M Yellon
Garrett J Gross

1

THE BIOLOGY OF K_{ATP} CHANNELS

NICHOLAS B STANDEN

Ion Channel Group, Department of Cell Physiology & Pharmacology, University of Leicester, P.O. Box 138, Leicester LE1 9HN, UK.

INTRODUCTION

ATP-sensitive potassium channels (K_{ATP} channels) provide a mechanism for linking membrane potassium permeability to cellular metabolism. They have important functions in the tissues of central importance to this book, cardiac muscle and systemic and coronary vascular smooth muscle. This chapter aims to present an overview of the biology of K_{ATP} channels with special reference to these tissues, with the emphasis on explanation rather than on a comprehensive review of what is already a very large literature. In this way, this chapter should provide a background for understanding the role of K_{ATP} channels in myocardial protection which forms the focus of this book.

K^+ channels are diverse, and this chapter will consider some of their general properties, before discussing the regulation of K_{ATP} channels by nucleotides and other factors, and outlining their pharmacology and their functions in the heart and vasculature. The biophysical properties and molecular structure of K_{ATP} channels are discussed briefly at the end of the chapter. For more detailed discussions of the various aspects of the cardiovascular K_{ATP} channels than is possible here, a number of recent reviews (1,2,3,4,5,6) may be of interest.

THE DIVERSITY OF POTASSIUM CHANNELS

Ion channels are proteins that span cell membranes and make them permeable to various physiological ions. Channel proteins are permeable to ions because they have an aqueous pore that runs right through the protein from the inside to the outside of the membrane, and through which ions can flow. Most channel proteins are selective; that is the pore allows one type of ion to pass through but excludes others. There are channel proteins selective for each of the major physiological ions (Na^+, Ca^{2+}, Cl^-), as well as non-selective cation channels, and an initial classification of channels is often made on the basis of their permeant ion. Thus potassium channels (K^+ channels) have a pore selective for K^+. In common with other types of channel, ion flow through K^+ channels is always passive, down the electrochemical gradient for potassium, and the aqueous pore leads to the rate of ion flow through the open channel protein being high, in the order of 10^6 to 10^7 ions per second. The ion flow through a channel carries electrical current, and the high rate of ion flow allows resolvable currents to be measured even from a single channel protein molecule. The electrophysiological technique that is used to measure these currents is the patch clamp, which can be used to record both from single channels and from whole cells, and has proved an extremely powerful method both for identifying channels and for studying their behaviour. Further discussion and excellent explanation of all aspects of ion channel physiology may be found in ref.(7), while their roles in cardiovascular medicine are discussed in ref. (8).

Ionic selectivity can be used to give a broad classification of ion channels, but there are several types of channel permeable to each ion species and K^+ channels are especially diverse. In common with other channels, the pore of most K^+ channels can be opened or closed ('gated') by a conformational change in the protein molecule. The various types of potassium channel share the property of selectivity to K^+, but differ for example in the factors that regulate channel opening and closing or in the rate at which K^+ flows through the open channel, usually expressed as the single channel conductance. These properties have been widely used to classify K^+ channels, and an outline of some of the main types is given in Table 1.

The main division on the basis of gating is between voltage-gated channels, whose opening and closing is primarily controlled by the membrane potential, and ligand-gated channels, where the major factor controlling gating is the binding of a chemical ligand, though ligand-gated channels often show some voltage sensitivity as well, which is not surprising for proteins that span the cell membrane and so are exposed to a high voltage field. As more channels are cloned, knowledge of their amino-acid sequences is increasingly providing another way to classify K^+ channels, and several molecular families are already known. For example the voltage-activated K_v superfamily of channels, derived originally from the cloning of the *Shaker* mutation of *Drosophila*, encompasses many related channels of both delayed rectifier and A-channel type. The differences in structure and physiological properties between different K^+ channels are often reflected in a different pharmacology. This is useful in assigning physiological functions to different K^+ channels, and also has practical value for therapeutic pharmacology.

Table 1 - Some types of K^+ channel

Channel	Abbreviations/ equivalent cloned channels	Gated by
Delayed rectifier	K_{DR}, K_v	Voltage
A-channel	K_A, K_{to}, K_v	Voltage
Inward rectifier	K_{IR}, IRK1	Spermine, Mg^{2+}, voltage, K^+
Ca^{2+}-activated	K_{Ca}, BK, SK	Calcium, (voltage)
ATP-sensitive	K_{ATP}	ATP_i, ADP_i
Muscarinic (m-channel)	K_{ACh}, GIRK	Acetylcholine

Thus ATP-sensitive K^+ channels have a K^+ selective pore, and intracellular ATP plays a role in their gating. Since their initial discovery in cardiac muscle in 1983 by Noma (9), K_{ATP} channels have been reported in a wide variety of tissues, including skeletal and smooth muscle, pancreatic beta cells, and certain central and peripheral neurones, and epithelial cells. Among these, the most work has been done in cardiac muscle and pancreatic beta or insulinoma cells, but there is already sufficient evidence to make it clear that K_{ATP} channels represent a family of channels, differing in their detailed properties between and maybe within tissues. Very recently, molecular biology is beginning to give indications as to the molecular structure, and this work is discussed briefly at the end of the chapter.

THE K^+ EQUILIBRIUM POTENTIAL HELPS UNDERSTAND THE FUNCTION OF K^+ CHANNELS

The general functions of K^+ channels can be predicted by understanding the concept of the potassium equilibrium potential, often abbreviated to E_K. K^+ is present inside cells at much higher concentration (around 155 mM), than in extracellular fluid (about 5 mM). This concentration gradient tends to cause K^+ to flow out of the cell. But as K^+ flows out it will set up a membrane potential, such that the inside of the cell becomes negative relative to the outside. This membrane potential represents an electrical gradient that opposes the efflux of K^+, and for given intracellular and extracellular concentrations of K^+ there will be a membrane potential at which the chemical and electrical forces exactly balance; the equilibrium potential for K^+, or E_K. E_K may be calculated from the K^+ concentrations using the Nernst equation:

$$E_K = RT/ZF \ln([K^+]_o/[K^+]_i) \qquad (1)$$

where E_K is the potassium equilibrium potential, $[K^+]_o$ and $[K^+]_i$ are the extracellular and intracellular concentrations of K^+ respectively, R is the Gas constant, T is the absolute temperature, Z is the valency (=1 for K^+), and F is Faraday's constant.

It is convenient to work out the constants at 37°C in millivolts (mV), and to convert from natural logarithms to $\log_{10}$, giving:

$$E_K = 61 mV \log_{10}([K^+]_o/[K^+]_i) \qquad (2)$$

Taking $[K^+]_i$ as 155 mM and $[K^+]_o$ as 5 mM gives E_K as -91 mV. Knowledge of E_K is useful because opening K^+ channels in a cell membrane will move the membrane potential towards E_K. Thus the functions of potassium channels include keeping the membrane potential of cells negative, producing the repolarizing (falling) phase of action potentials, and providing a mechanism for hyperpolarization.

SINGLE CHANNELS AND CURRENT FLOW IN WHOLE CELLS

K_{ATP} channels were first identified at the single channel level, and because excised membrane patches allow manipulation of the solution bathing the cytoplasmic face of the channel, many subsequent experimental studies of K_{ATP} channels have used single channel recording. However the final functional effects of these, as other, channels occur as a result of the activity of the entire population of channels in a whole cell membrane, and there are also many studies of whole cells or intact tissues. It is useful, therefore, to consider how the current flowing through such a population of channels is related to the behaviour of its individual members. We are concerned only with two properties of each channel; whether or not it is open, and the rate at which ions flow through if it is. Over a period of time, the proportion of that time which a channel spends open will give its chance of being open, usually called open probability, or P_{open}. The rate at which ions go through the open channel is given by the single channel current, normally represented by i and expressed in picoamperes. (One picoampere, 1 pA, equals 10^{-12} amps and corresponds to a flow of 6.2×10^6 monovalent ions per second).

The mean current through a population of N channels, $\bar{I}$, will simply be given by

$$\bar{I} = N.i.P_{open} \qquad (3)$$

The number of channels in the cell should be constant, at least in the short term. The single channel current, i, depends on the conductance of the channel, a measure of how easily ions can pass through, a property fixed by the molecular architecture of the channel pore, and on the membrane potential, since this controls the electrochemical gradient for K^+. Thus processes that control or modulate channel activity usually do so changing P_{open}. Provided that membrane potential (and so i) does not change, eqn (3) also means that a plot of P_{open} against, for example ATP concentration (Figure 1), will also represent the ATP dependence of the number of *open* channels in a whole cell.

K_{ATP} CHANNELS ARE CLOSED BY INTRACELLULAR ATP

K_{ATP} channels were first identified in membrane patches excised from cardiac myocytes as K^+ channels that were inhibited when ATP was applied to the cytoplasmic face of the membrane (9). This defining property is illustrated in Figure 1, which shows the relation between channel open probability and the ATP concentration bathing the intracellular face of a patch of membrane from a cardiac muscle cell. As [ATP] is increased, P_{open} falls, with half inhibition occurring at 25 μM ATP. The concentration dependence of channel closure by ATP can be fitted with a Hill curve, with values for the Hill coefficient in cardiac muscle usually around 2 (4), though values between 1 and 6 have been reported (10). It has been suggested that there are one, two or more binding sites for ATP on the K_{ATP} channel (1,3).

K_{ATP} channel closure does not require hydrolysis of ATP. ATP is effective in the absence of Mg^{2+}, and non-hydrolysable analogues of ATP, for example AMP-PNP, are effective in causing channel closure (5). This suggests that ATP simply binds to a site or sites on the channel protein to cause closure, and estimates of the rate of ATP binding can be obtained from single channel kinetics (12). The site is clearly intracellular, since ATP is ineffective from outside the cell. In addition, inhibition by ATP shows little or no voltage-dependence, although the ATP molecule is negatively charged, suggesting that the site is on a domain of the channel which does not experience the voltage field across the cell membrane (4), though surface charge may affect the local ATP concentration at its binding site (13).

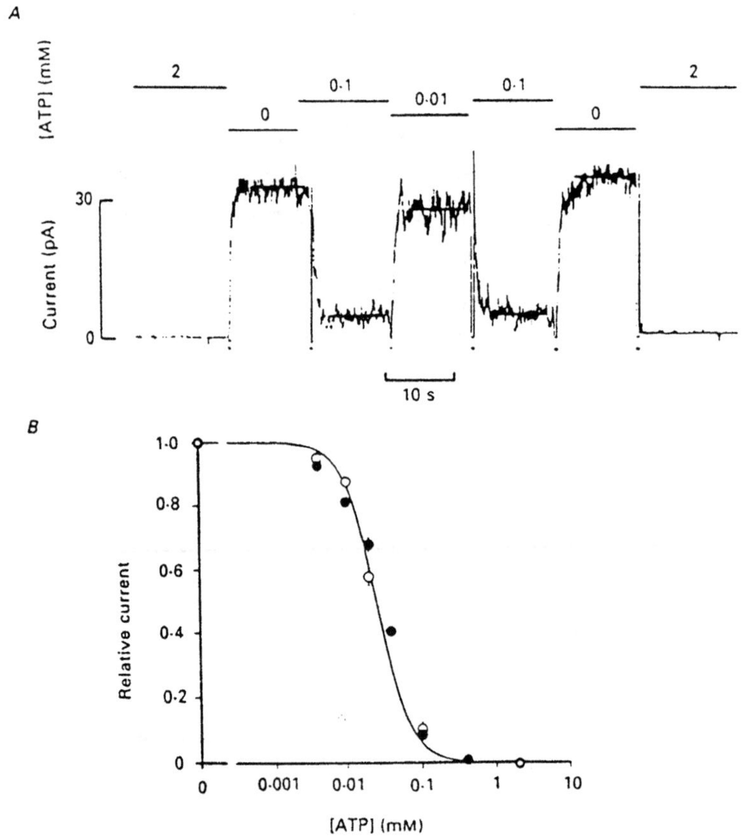

Figure 1. K_{ATP} channel closure by ATP. A, The current recorded using patch clamp from an inside out patch excised from rat ventricular muscle as the internal [ATP] was varied between 0 and 2 mM as shown above. The patch contained about 20 channels. B, The ATP-dependence of the channel open probability. The relative current (ordinate) gives a measure of P_{open}, so that 1.0 corresponds to the maximal P_{open} in the absence of ATP, close to 1 in these experiments. Open and filled circles show measurements in zero and 0.5 mM Mg^{2+}, respectively. Reproduced from (11) with permission.

Further information about the ATP binding site(s) of the K_{ATP} channel can be obtained from the effects of other nucleotides in causing channel inhibition. ADP, AMP, GTP, CTP, UTP and ITP all cause inhibition, but are less potent than ATP itself. Such findings suggest that the site can recognise all regions of the ATP molecule; in cardiac muscle it appears, however, not to distinguish between ATP and MgATP (1,5; Figure 1).

The sensitivity of the K_{ATP} channel to intracellular ATP immediately suggested a role in linking membrane K^+ permeability to cellular metabolism (9). Two kinds of difficulties arose with the idea that ATP alone might regulate channel activity, however. First, the ATP concentration that causes half-inhibition is usually found to be in the range 10-100 μM, suggesting that, in the absence of other regulatory factors, very few K_{ATP} channels would be expected to be open at the normal intracellular [ATP] of around 5 mM. Secondly, the intracellular ATP concentration is well buffered and so is very resistant to metabolic changes. For example, in hearts exposed to cyanide cardiac action potential shortening occurs before a significant decrease in ATP concentration (14). The first problem may simply reflect the fact that, as will be discussed later when we consider the functions of K_{ATP} channels in cardiovascular tissues, rather few K_{ATP} channels out of the total cellular population may need to open to exert significant effects on the cell. The second problem, that ATP changes little until metabolism is severely compromised, has led to a number of suggestions as to how the K_{ATP} channel may be regulated (1,5,15,16). It is possible that the submembrane ATP concentration, which is what should control the K_{ATP} channel, might be different from, or change more than that in the bulk cytoplasm. It has also been suggested that a population of K_{ATP} channels may have varying sensitivities to ATP, or that glycolyis may preferentially regulate their activity. Finally, there is substantial evidence that other intracellular factors in addition to ATP control K_{ATP} channel activity, and we will now consider some of these.

OTHER INTRACELLULAR METABOLIC REGULATORS MODULATE THE ATP SENSITIVITY OF K_{ATP} CHANNELS

Intracellular factors that affect K_{ATP} channels of cardiac muscle include ADP, lactate, and intracellular pH. Intracellular ADP, in the presence of Mg^{2+}, has been shown to reduce channel inhibition by ATP, an effect that apparently depends on MgADP competing with ATP for its binding site (5,17). Intracellular ADP rises rapidly during hypoxia or ischaemia, and it may be that the K_{ATP} channel is effectively regulated by the ADP/ATP ratio rather than by ATP alone (13). Intracellular pH, which also changes rapidly in the anoxic heart (5) has also been shown to affect cardiac K_{ATP} channels, a fall in pH leading to decrease in ATP sensitivity and so in channel inhibition by ATP (11,18). The effect occurs over the range pH 7.6-6.0, and has been modelled on the basis that protonation of sites on the channel protein may prevent the binding of ATP to its inhibitory site (12). In addition, intracellular lactate, which also accumulates in ischaemia, has been reported to activate cardiac K_{ATP} channels (19,20).

All the regulators described above depend on cellular metabolism and so will contribute to the metabolic regulation of the channel. In addition, all these factors appear to exert their effects by causing a shift in the ATP-inhibition curve so that they reduce channel inhibition by ATP. Thus a rise in ADP or lactate concentration, or a fall in pH, will cause an increase in K_{ATP} channel open probability at a fixed ATP concentration. These factors may all be expected to change both to a greater extent and more rapidly in response to a change in cellular metabolic status than does ATP itself. In this way, ATP may be seen as a background regulator of the channel, binding to the channel protein to set a low background P_{open}, against which changes in other regulators control channel activity by altering the affinity for ATP and so the degree of channel inhibition.

K_{ATP} CHANNELS CAN BE MODULATED BY G-PROTEIN COUPLED RECEPTORS

In addition to regulation by metabolic factors acting from the inside of the cell, it is clear that the activity of K_{ATP} channels of both cardiac and smooth muscle can be modulated by transmitters that activate membrane receptors linked to G-proteins.

In cardiac ventricular myocytes, extracellular adenosine activates a whole cell K_{ATP} current (21; Figure 2). In membrane patches excised from cardiac muscle, G-protein activation by GTPγs or AlF^{4-} applied to the cytoplasmic face of the patch leads to K_{ATP} channel activation, as do the preactivated G-protein α-subunits $G_{\alpha i\text{-}1}$, $G_{\alpha i\text{-}2}$ (21,22). GTP applied to the cytoplasmic face only causes activation if adenosine or acetylcholine is present in the extracellular solution (21,22,23). The adenosine receptor involved appears to be of the A_1 type. These studies suggest that adenosine, binding to an A_1 receptor, activates K_{ATP} channels by way of a membrane-delimited pathway involving the α-subunit of the pertussis toxin sensitive G-protein G_i (Figure 2). Acetylcholine appears to be able to activate the same pathway by way of a muscarinic receptor (24). It has recently been shown that these G-protein activation pathways antagonize K_{ATP} channel inhibition by ATP, so that they appear to act in a similar way to the metabolic regulators discussed above, that is by modulating the sensitivity of the K_{ATP} channel to inhibition by ATP (22,23).

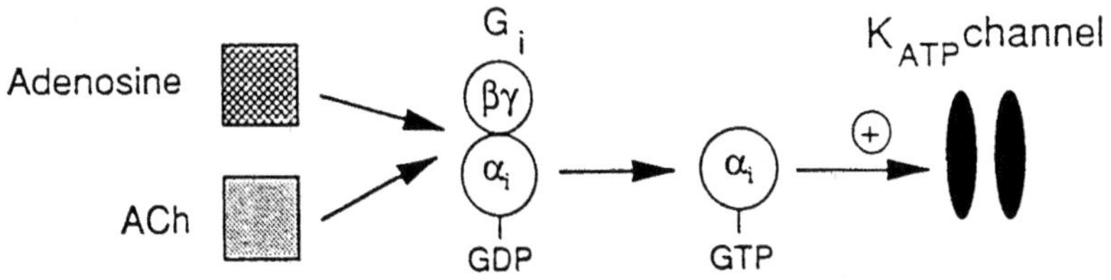

Figure 2. Mechanism of activation of cardiac K_{ATP} channels by G protein. Both adenosine binding to A_1 receptors and acetylcholine at muscarinic receptors can activate the pertussis toxin sensitive G-protein G_i. The α subunit activates K_{ATP} in a membrane-delimited pathway. The βγ subunit can activate K_{ACh}, a pathway that may be confined to atrial cells (24).

Receptor modulation of K_{ATP} channel activity has also been demonstrated in vascular smooth muscle (Figure 3). In coronary arteries, adenosine A_1 receptors activate K_{ATP} channels by a mechanism that may be similar to that described in cardiac muscle (25). There is also evidence that transmitters which activate receptors coupled to adenylyl cyclase activate K_{ATP} channels, suggesting that phosphorylation by protein kinase A (PKA) may lead to K_{ATP} channel activation. The transmitters include calcitonin gene-related peptide (CGRP) and β_1 adrenergic agonists, and are discussed later when the involvement of K_{ATP} channels in vasodilation is considered. The involvement of the PKA pathway has been most clearly demonstrated for the action of CGRP on cells from mesenteric artery, where the catalytic subunit of PKA has been shown to activate K_{ATP} channels (26). In addition, nitric oxide (EDRF) and atrial natriuretic factor have also both been proposed to activate K_{ATP} channels in some vascular tissues. Since both increase cyclic GMP levels, it is also possible that K_{ATP} channels can be activated by cGMP or cGMP-dependent protein kinase.

Several vasoconstrictor agents are known to activate protein kinase C (PKC), and in cultured coronary arterial smooth muscle vasopressin, angiotensin II, and endothelin have all been reported to inhibit K_{ATP} channels (27,28,29), suggesting that the channel might be inhibited by phosphorylation by PKC. Such a pathway has been shown to be involved in K_{ATP} channel inhibition by muscarinic agonists in bladder smooth muscle (30), but it is worth noting that K_{ATP} inhibition by PKC linked vasconstrictors has yet to be demonstrated in freshly isolated, rather than cultured, coronary smooth muscle.

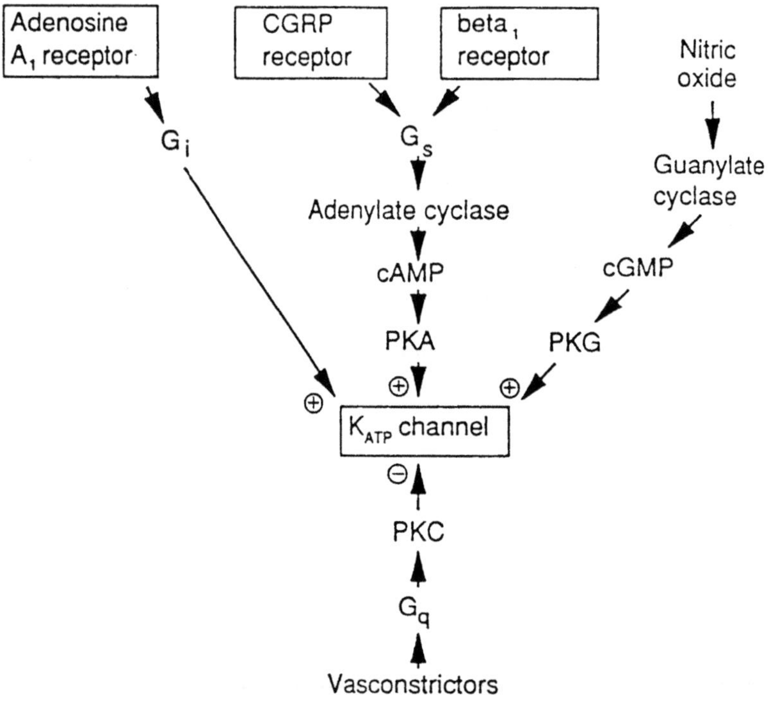

Figure 3. Pathways that may be involved in transmitter modulation of the K_{ATP} channel of arterial smooth muscle.

NUCLEOTIDES ALSO MAINTAIN CHANNEL ACTIVITY

As well as binding to K_{ATP} channels to cause inhibition (as for ATP), or to modulate this effect (ADP), intracellular nucleotides are also necessary for the maintenance of K_{ATP} channels in a functional state so that they are able to open in response to changes in ATP or other regulators. Both MgATP and nucleoside diphosphates appear to play roles in this maintenance of channel activity.

When a membrane patch is excised into an ATP-free or low ATP solution, K_{ATP} channel activity is observed to decline with time after excision (Figure 4), a phenomenon generally called run down (31,32). Run down is accentuated by Ca^{2+}

or Mg^{2+} in the internal solution, leading to the suggestion that it may involve Ca^{2+}-dependent phosphatases, though it has so far proved insensitive to phosphatase inhibitors (33,34). In some preparations, treatment with trypsin has been found to slow run down, suggesting that trypsin may remove or alter some regulatory protein associated with the channel (5,34). Internal MgATP can restore channel activity after run down, so that ATP does not only inhibit K_{ATP} channels, but also maintains them in an activatable state. Unlike channel inhibition, reactivation after run down is only seen with MgATP, and non-hydrolysable ATP analogues are ineffective (35). It has therefore often been proposed that maintenance of channel activity involves ATP hydrolysis and phosphorylation of the K_{ATP} channel or an associated protein (e.g. 32). However, Furukawa et al. (35) recently found that inhibitors of serine/threonine protein kinases did not suppress channel reactivation by MgATP, and therefore conclude that, though ATP hydrolysis appears to be important, protein phosphorylation may not be involved in reactivation.

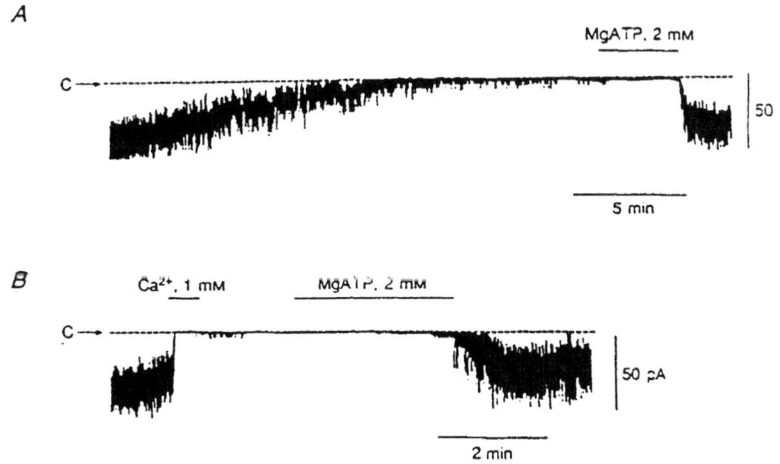

Figure 4. K_{ATP} channel run down and reactivation by MgATP. A, Channel run down in a multi-channel inside-out patch excised from a guinea-pig ventricular cell. C shows the level with all channels closed. After excision, channel activity ran down with time, but was reactivated by exposure to MgATP. The restored activity is seen after removal of MgATP, when channel inhibition by ATP is removed. B, Run down occurs faster in the presence of internal Ca^{2+}, but activity is still restored by MgATP. Reproduced from (35) with permission.

Nucleoside diphosphates (NDPs) also seem to have a function in maintaining K_{ATP} channel activity. As well as reducing channel inhibition by ATP, NDPs have been reported to activate K_{ATP} channels in the absence of ATP in both cardiac and vascular smooth muscle (11,17,39). Like ATP, they are able to restore channel activity after run down, and similarly require the presence of Mg^{2+} to exert this effect (36). Uridine diphosphate is the most effective in cardiac muscle, followed by inosine, cytidine and guanosine diphosphates. This action of nucleoside diphosphates appears to be separate from their effects in reducing channel inhibition by ATP since channels reactivated with nucleoside diphosphates do not show an altered ATP affinity (36). Thus the K_{ATP} channel may have a Mg^{2+} dependent binding site for NDPs which can maintain channel activity or reactivate run down channels (5,36). Terzic et al. (37) have proposed that the K_{ATP} channel can switch between a run down state where NDPs can activate it and an active state where NDPs antagonize inhibition by ATP, so that the effect of NDPs on the channel is regulated by an MgATP-dependent reaction.

In smooth muscle cells from portal vein or mesenteric artery GDP or other NDPs were found to activate glibenclamide-sensitive channels, while depletion of ATP alone had little effect (38,39,40). Activation was Mg^{2+} dependent, and the NDP activated current was reduced by about 64% by 1 mM ATP. Beech et al. (39) have referred to these channels as K_{NDP} channels to emphasize the role played by NDPs in their regulation. It has, of course, been quite widely suggested that changes in intracellular ATP concentration *per se* are not the major regulator of the K_{ATP} channel in many tissues (e.g.1,2).

PHARMACOLOGICAL BLOCKERS AND OPENERS OF K_{ATP} CHANNELS

The pharmacological properties of K_{ATP} channels have been central to the elucidation of their functions in cardiovascular tissues. This section will not attempt to provide a comprehensive review of K_{ATP} pharmacology (see 41,42 for reviews), but rather to emphasize aspects which have been important for beginning to understand the physiological relevance of these channels.

Blockers

K_{ATP} channels are blocked by antidiabetic sulphonylurea drugs. Glibenclamide (glyburide) has been the most widely used of these, and much of the evidence for the involvement of K_{ATP} channels in physiological processes relies on the demonstration of sensitivity to glibenclamide. Glibenclamide has been used to block K_{ATP} channels in cardiovascular tissues at concentrations in the range 10 nM - 100 μM. It has been reported to be effective in heart at 0.1 - 10 μM (43,44), and a K_i as low as 6 nM has been reported in cardiac muscle (45), though it has been suggested that K_{ATP} channels may become much less sensitive to glibenclamide during extreme metabolic stress (46). In vascular smooth muscle (portal vein) cells K_i values of 25 and 200 nM have been measured for the effects of glibenclamide on K_{ATP} current induced by GDP and cromakalim respectively (39). In these cells glibenclamide at high concentrations (K_i = 100 μM) also inhibited a different K^+ channel, the delayed rectifier. Glibenclamide has not been reported to block other types of K^+ channel in cardiovascular tissues, so that it appears to be selective for K_{ATP} in these tissues at concentrations up to about 10 μM. Other sulphonylureas can also block K_{ATP} channels, but only tolbutamide has been used widely, and is much less potent than glibenclamide. A chemically different type of blocker that may also be selective for K_{ATP} channels is 5-hydroxydecanoate (55).

K_{ATP} channels are also sensitive to several blockers that affect most types of K^+ channel, though with varying potencies. These include tetraethylammonium ions (TEA^+), 4-aminopyridine, phencyclidine, and barium and caesium ions. Several of these are charged, and because their action is voltage-sensitive are thought to block within the channel pore, a structure which is quite highly conserved among different K^+ channels. These blockers provide interesting information about the properties of K_{ATP} channels and their relation to other K^+ channels, but because of their lack of selectivity, are of less use in assigning physiological functions to the channel.

Openers

Table 2 - Drugs that open K_{ATP} channels

Opener	Derived from
Cromakalim, Levcromakalim	benzopyran
Pinacidil	pyridylcyanoguanidine
Nicorandil	nicotinamide
RP 49356, Aprikalim	carbothiamide
Minoxidil	pyrimidine
Diazoxide	benzothiadiazine

A chemically diverse group of drugs (Table 2) activates K_{ATP} channels. These are generally referred to as K^+ channel openers or KCOs since all the first K^+ channel opening drugs had K_{ATP} channels as their target. Recently, however, openers of Ca^{2+}-activated K^+ channels have been reported, so that it may be more appropriate to refer to those that target K_{ATP} as K_{ATP} channel openers. These drugs, and their effects on the vasculature and heart have been reviewed recently (47,48,49) and the aim here will be just to provide an overview of their actions.

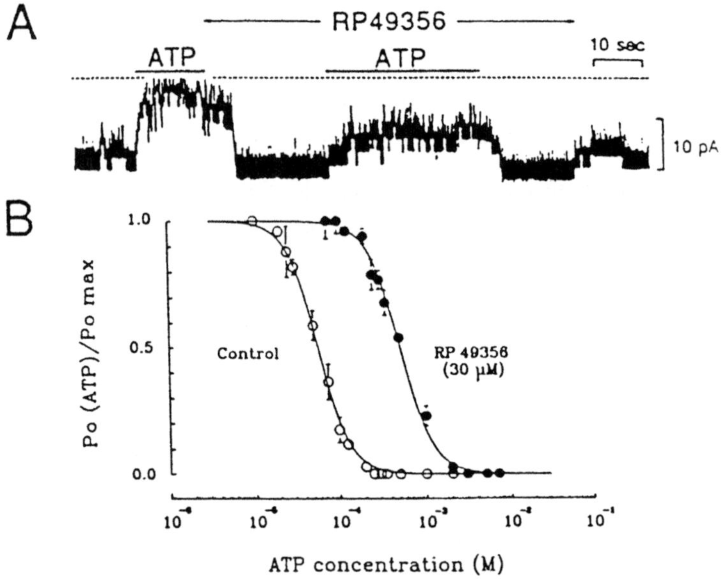

Figure 5. The effect of a K_{ATP} channel opener on cardiac K_{ATP} channels. A, Recording of channel activity in a patch excised from a guinea-pig ventricular myocyte. Channel openings caused inward current, and the dotted line shows the zero current level. ATP (100 μM) inhibited channel activity less in the presence of the opener RP 49356 (30 μM). B, RP 49356 shifted the relation between channel P_{open} and [ATP] to higher ATP concentrations. Reproduced from (50) with permission.

K_{ATP} channel openers have been shown to activate K_{ATP} currents in smooth muscle cells isolated from a number of tissues. They generally act at low (nM to low μM) concentrations, and, because the resting membrane potential is distant from E_K cause substantial hyperpolarization and so relaxation. They are therefore potent vasodilators and have been shown to increase blood flow in several tissues, mimicking the natural role of K_{ATP} channels in response to hypoxia or endogenous vasodilators. K_{ATP} channel openers appear to be more effective under conditions where K_{ATP} activation is already enhanced, as with reduced intracellular ATP or in hypoxia, and in this way may have the useful property of targeting ischaemic tissue.

K_{ATP} channel openers appear to be less potent in cardiac muscle than in smooth muscle. Thus in normoxic cardiac muscle, concentrations that can produce substantial vasodilation have no detectable effect on the resting or action potential of cardiac muscle, though such concentrations may be cardioprotective. At higher concentrations (10-1000 μM), K_{ATP} channel openers activate measurable K_{ATP} currents in isolated cardiac myocytes, and progressively shorten the cardiac action potential. However they cause only slight depolarization, since the resting potential of cardiac muscle is already quite near to E_K. Figure 5 illustrates a common property of the action of K_{ATP} channel openers; the ATP-inhibition curve is shifted to higher ATP concentrations, so that it appears that the openers reduce K_{ATP} channel sensitivity for ATP (48,49). In this way, their effects may be thought of as similar to the endogenous metabolic regulators ADP, pH, and lactate. Under some conditions, however, K_{ATP} channel openers can also open channels in the absence of ATP (49). The consequence of the interaction of openers and ATP concentration, and probably also of a synergistic action of openers and the other metabolic regulators described above, is that K_{ATP} channel openers are much more potent in the metabolically compromised myocardium than in normoxia.

FUNCTIONS OF K_{ATP} CHANNELS IN CARDIAC MUSCLE

In cardiac muscle the proposed functions of K_{ATP} channels relate to the response of the tissue to hypoxia or ischaemia. The channels are involved in the shortening of the cardiac action potential and the increase in K^+ efflux seen under these conditions and, presumably through these effects, can act to protect the ischaemic myocardium. As well as immediate protection during ischaemia and reperfusion, there is good evidence that K_{ATP} channels are involved in protection against the effects of subsequent periods of ischaemia; the phenomenon known as preconditioning which is discussed in Chapter 4.

Hypoxia or ischaemia leads to a progressive decline in the duration of the cardiac action potential (Figure 6), and eventually failure of the action potential and of contraction. Noma (9), when he first identified the K_{ATP} channel, suggested that its role might be to cause this action potential shortening in hypoxia, so reducing cardiac energy consumption and protecting the hypoxiC heart. Subsequent studies have confirmed the role of the channel in action potential shortening. In both isolated cells and intact hearts the reduction in action potential duration is reduced or abolished by glibenclamide, tolbutamide, or 5-hydroxydecanoate, blockers of the K_{ATP} channel (51,52,53,54,55,56; Figure 6). Intracellular delivery of ATP by way of a patch pipette to increase $[ATP]_i$ and so inhibit K_{ATP} channels has also been shown to partially restore the action potential duration (57). Further, drugs such as pinacidil that activate the K_{ATP} channel reduce the duration of the cardiac action potential at high concentrations, and also speed the time course of action potential shortening in ischaemia (53,58).

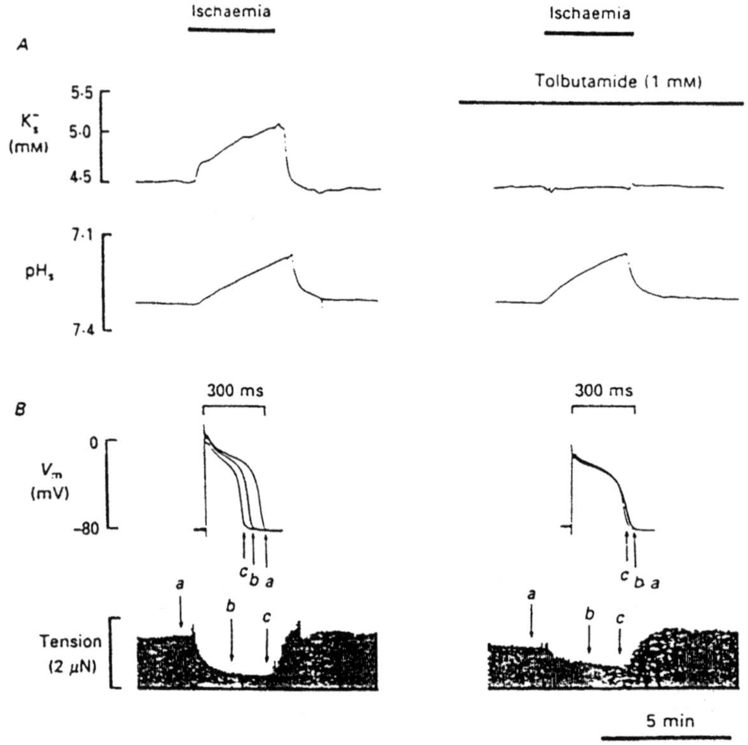

Figure 6. K^+ efflux and shortening of the cardiac action potential in ischaemia. A, the rise in extracellular K^+ measured with a K^+ electrode just outside a Purkinje fibre exposed to simulated ischaemia. The right hand record shows the abolition of the K^+ efflux by tolbutamide, while the fall in extracellular pH is unaffected. B, ischaemia leads to a progressive shortening of the action potential and decline in contractile force, and this effect is attenuated by tolbutamide. Reproduced from (51) with permission.

Ischaemia leads to a rapid rise in extracellular K^+ concentration, so depolarizing the cardiac muscle. This may contribute to the reduction in action potential duration and failure of contractile function. The increased $[K^+]_o$ results from an increased efflux of K^+ from the ischaemic myocardium, and at least part of this K^+ efflux occurs through K_{ATP} channels. Blockade of K_{ATP} channels reduces extracellular K^+ accumulation (51,54,56,58), while their activation with nicorandil can increase the rise in $[K^+]_o$ seen during ischaemia (59).

The effects described above suggest that K_{ATP} channel activation in ischaemia accentuates action potential shortening and so will lead to earlier failure of the action potential and contraction. These actions are thought to be cytoprotective because they reduce Ca^{2+} entry and so Ca^{2+} overload, but the mechanisms underlying cytoprotection are certainly not completely understood. It has also been argued that the action potential shortening and K^+ accumulation resulting from K_{ATP} channel activation might increase the likelihood of cardiac arrhythmias, while alternatively it has been suggested that the more rapid action potential failure and reduction in Ca^{2+} overload in ischaemic regions might be antiarrhythmogenic. These issues are outside the scope of the present chapter, but are considered in Chapter 5 of this book.

K_{ATP} channels are present at high density in the membrane of ventricular cells, so that there are several thousand channels per cell. It has been shown that opening of less than 1% of these channels is sufficient to produce the action potential shortening seen in hypoxia (1,10). Thus the K_{ATP} channels of cardiac muscle may work over a range where their P_{open} is very low, but of course still sensitive to ATP, and to the modulation of this sensitivity by ADP, pH, lactate, and adenosine. In ischaemia, these factors combine to raise P_{open} by a small amount, which is nevertheless sufficient to produce the effects on action potential duration and K^+ efflux described above.

K_{ATP} CHANNELS PROVIDE A PATHWAY FOR VASODILATION IN VASCULAR SMOOTH MUSCLE

K_{ATP} channels of arterial smooth muscle provide a mechanism for vasodilation in response to changes in metabolic state (for example in hypoxia or ischaemia) and to a number of endogenous transmitters. Activation of K_{ATP} channels is transduced into a vasorelaxing response by the hyperpolarization that it causes. The amplitude of whole-cell currents activated by maximal concentrations of K_{ATP} opening drugs

suggests that there are only a few hundred K_{ATP} channels in a vascular smooth muscle cell. Nevertheless, because vascular smooth muscle cells have a high input resistance, corresponding to a low level of channel activity in the resting membrane, activation of a few channels can have substantial effects on membrane potential (60). Thus it seems that, as for cardiac muscle, K_{ATP} channels normally operate at very low open probabilities at physiological concentrations of nucleotides. In the coronary circulation there is evidence that the resting open probability of K_{ATP} channels may be sufficient for them to contribute to the maintenance of the resting membrane potential in the absence of vasodilator influences, raising the additional possibility that channel closure could play a part in vasoconstrictor responses.
The membrane potential of vascular smooth muscle, in the range -30 to -70 mV, is considerably more depolarized than the equilibrium potential for K^+, around -90 mV (60,61). Thus opening of K^+ channels will cause the smooth muscle cell membrane potential to hyperpolarize towards E_K. The membrane potential regulates calcium entry into the cell through voltage-dependent calcium channels which are very sensitive to membrane potential in the physiological range, with a 5 mV hyperpolarization causing an approximately 2.7 fold decrease in the channel open probability (60). In addition, membrane hyperpolarization may also reduce inositol 1,4,5-trisphosphate mediated intracellular calcium release (62,63). Both effects will lead to a decrease in intracellular Ca^{2+} concentration, thus reducing contractile tone by way of myosin light chain kinase and the interaction of actin and myosin. Thus hyperpolarization leads to relaxation of vascular smooth muscle and so vasodilation.

Metabolic regulation of blood flow.

Blood flow is closely linked to metabolic demand in several regional circulations including the coronary, skeletal muscle and cerebral circulations. In these circulations hypoxia increases blood flow, and the response to hypoxia could occur in two general ways. First, cellular activity can cause local hypoxia, making the environment of the smooth muscle of the vasculature hypoxic. This would increase the level of nucleoside diphosphates, and perhaps decrease $[ATP]_i$, leading to activation of K_{ATP} channels, causing smooth muscle membrane hyperpolarization and vasodilation. It is also possible that a fall in pO_2 may affect channel activity without changing intracellular nucleoside phosphates, by way of an oxygen sensing mechanism such as has been proposed for cells of the carotid body. Secondly, cellular activity in the tissue surrounding the blood vessel will result in release of metabolites such as protons, adenosine, and K^+ into the extracellular space. Several of these metabolites are potent vasodilators, relaxing vascular smooth muscle by a number of mechanisms which may include activation of K_{ATP} channels, as for example by adenosine. Thus metabolites will act locally to dilate blood vessels, increasing blood supply. Extracellular and intracellular pathways will converge at the level of the K_{ATP} channel to promote metabolic vasodilation. A good example of this may be found in the coronary circulation, where there is evidence that both adenosine and hypoxia cause coronary vasodilation by activating K_{ATP} channels.

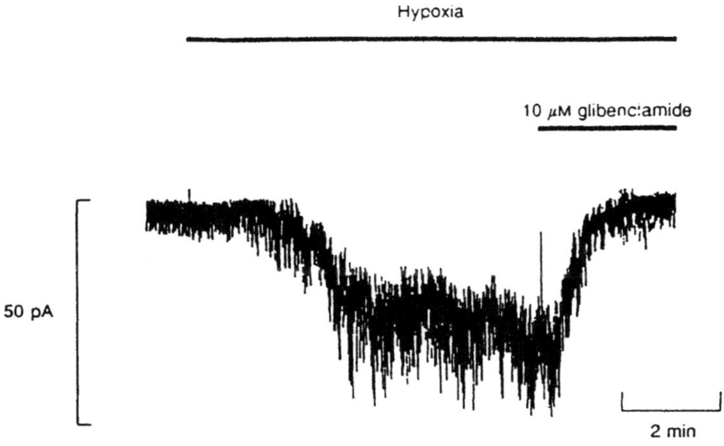

Figure 7. K_{ATP} channel activation by hypoxia in a coronary arterial myocyte. The record shows the K^+ current elicited by superfusion of an isolated myocyte from a pig small coronary artery with a hypoxic solution (pO_2 25-40 mmHg), and its inhibition by glibenclamide. The recording was made using the perforated patch whole-cell recording technique. Reproduced from (69) with permission.

Evidence for the involvement of K_{ATP} channels in hypoxic vasodilation comes from the observation that such vasodilation is blocked by K_{ATP} channel inhibition with glibenclamide in coronary, skeletal muscle and cerebral vascular beds (64,65,66,67,68). The mechanisms have been most extensively studied in the coronary circulation. At the level of coronary arterial myocytes both adenosine and hypoxia cause K_{ATP} channel activation (25,69, Figure 7), and in the intact, perfused guinea-pig heart vasodilation to either adenosine or hypoxia is glibenclamide-sensitive (70). Early hypoxic vasodilation is not reversed by adenosine receptor antagonists in this system, so that this phase may therefore be a direct consequence of decreased tissue pO_2, resulting in activation of K_{ATP} channels through metabolic changes in coronary smooth muscle, rather than a secondary response to adenosine released by the hypoxic myocardium (70). However the late phase of hypoxic vasodilation in the same preparation may involve adenosine and prostaglandins (71), while adenosine release seems to play a significant role in K_{ATP} channel activation during hypoxic vasodilation in the isolated rabbit heart (66).

K_{ATP} channels also appear to be involved in the autoregulation of coronary and cerebral blood flow. Autoregulation is characterised by an ability to maintain constant blood flow when perfusion pressure changes. Glibenclamide abolished coronary autoregulation in anaesthetised dogs, and also prevented the dilation of small coronary arteries to reductions in perfusion pressure (72,73). Cerebral autoregulation has also been reported to be disrupted by glibenclamide, and here the activation of K_{ATP} channels by CGRP may be important in autoregulation (74).

In certain vascular beds, K_{ATP} channels may make a significant contribution to the resting membrane potential, and so to the basal vascular tone under normoxic conditions. Such a role has received experimental support in the coronary circulation, where glibenclamide increases coronary tone *in vivo* (75,76) and depolarizes coronary smooth muscle (77). Involvement of K_{ATP} channels in the resting membrane potential has also been proposed in mesenteric and pulmonary arteries (78,79).

Vasodilation in response to endogenous transmitters.

In addition to regulating blood flow in response to metabolic changes, K_{ATP} channels of vascular smooth muscle provide important targets for a number of endogenous hyperpolarizing vasodilators. Some of these have been mentioned above in the context of channel modulation by G-proteins. The evidence for K_{ATP} involvement in the hyperpolarizing actions of these vasodilators ranges from measurement of K_{ATP} channel activation in single cells to demonstrations of glibenclamide-sensitive vasodilation. Vasodilators that may activate K_{ATP} include adenosine, CGRP, VIP, adrenaline, ADP, prostacyclin, nitric oxide, EDHF and atrial natriuretic factor (25,26,65,66,67,70,74,80,81,82,83,84). Thus an important role of K_{ATP} in vascular smooth muscle is to provide a mechanism for the vasodilator action of these agents by acting as a target for their receptor-mediated pathways. It is important to note that these vasodilators can also relax arteries by K^+ channel-independent mechanisms, so that K_{ATP} channels provide one pathway for their actions, and that the relative importance of this pathway clearly differs between different vascular beds. The possibility that K_{ATP} channel inhibition may contribute to the action of some vasoconstrictors has been considered above in the context of possible inhibition by protein kinase C.

A SUMMARY OF THE ROLE OF K_{ATP} CHANNELS IN THE ISCHAEMIC HEART

The cardiovascular functions described above combine to provide an integrated response to hypoxia in the ischaemic heart, summarized in Figure 8. Decreased oxygen delivery will compromise the metabolism of cardiac muscle, leading to increased intracellular ADP and lactate, decreased pH, possibly a fall in ATP, and release of adenosine into the extracellular space. These intracellular factors, together with activation of A_1 receptors by adenosine will activate cardiac K_{ATP} channels, leading to action potential shortening, decreased calcium entry and contractile force, and release of K^+. In smooth muscle cells of the coronary arteries, local hypoxia may also activate K_{ATP} channels through a rise in intracellular NDPs and a fall in ATP, and the channels will also be activated by adenosine. K_{ATP} activation will result in hyperpolarization and vasodilation, increasing blood flow and so oxygen delivery to the region. Activation of inward rectifier K^+ channels by the rise in extracellular K^+ may contribute to the vasodilation (85). The final results of K_{ATP} activation will be to reduce cardiac energy consumption, and to restore blood flow as far as possible, both of which effects should contribute to protection of the myocardium.

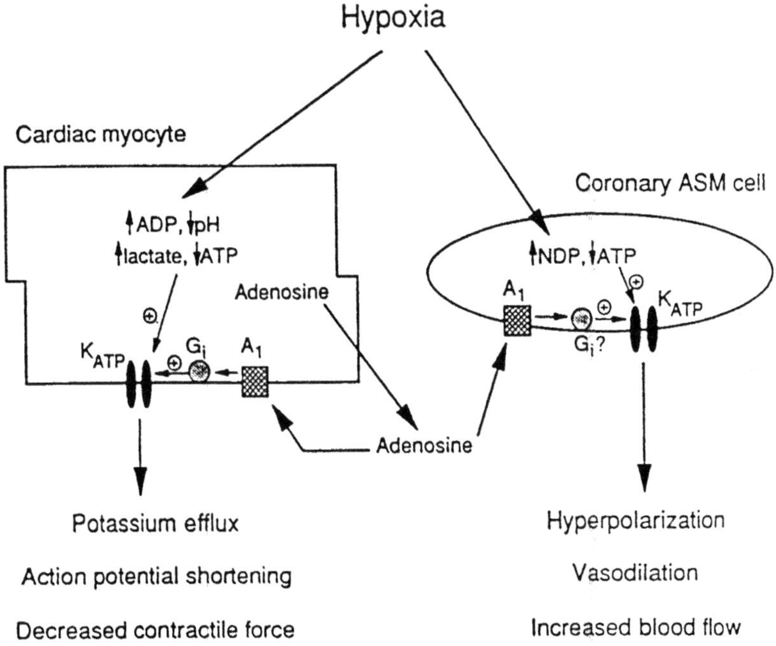

Figure 8. The involvement of K_{ATP} channels in the responses of cardiac muscle and coronary smooth muscle cells to ischaemia.

BIOPHYSICAL PROPERTIES OF K_{ATP} CHANNELS

High selectivity for K^+ is a general property of K^+ channels, reflecting the relatively highly conserved structure of the pore region among different channel types, and K_{ATP} channels are also highly selective for K^+, with the permeability to K^+ being at least 60-fold higher than that to Na^+ (2,31). The reported unitary conductance of K_{ATP} channels varies, contributing to the evidence that K_{ATP} channels form a family, rather than a single type of channel. Since conductance varies with $[K^+]$, it is also important to compare conductances in equivalent external and internal K^+ concentrations; the most convenient is normally symmetrical high K^+ (120-150 mM). Under these conditions, cardiac K_{ATP} channels (1,4,5) have conductances around 80-90 pS (a siemen is a reciprocal Ohm, and 1 pS or picosiemen = 10^{-12} S). In smooth muscle, K_{ATP} channels of both small (20-50 ps) and large (100-260 pS) conductance have been reported from single channel studies, though most studies of activation by K_{ATP} channel openers, metabolic inhibition, or endogenous vasodilators suggest the involvement of small conductance channels (6). Under physiological conditions, K_{ATP} channels also show moderate inward rectification, so that inward K^+ currents are larger than outward currents. This rectification is caused by intracellular Mg^{2+} and to a lesser extent Na^+, which act as voltage-dependent blockers of the channel from the inside (4,86).

The P_{open} of K_{ATP} channels shows little voltage or time dependence (1,2,3). However, their single channel kinetics are clearly complex, with channel openings being grouped in bursts separated by longer closed periods. ATP affects these kinetics in several ways, it shortens openings, shortens the durations of bursts of openings, and increases the proportion of channel closures that are of very long duration .

INDICATIONS ABOUT THE MOLECULAR STRUCTURE OF K_{ATP} CHANNELS

Both voltage-activated (K_v family) and inward rectifier (IRK family) K^+ channels form as tetramers of subunits but are distinguished by the K_v channel subunits having six membrane-spanning regions while inward rectifier subunits have just two (87,88). K_{ATP} channels appear to belong to the inward rectifier family. This family comprises both strong inward rectifiers like IRK1, which have recently been shown to rectify strongly because of block by intracellular spermine (89,90), and channels which rectify more weakly, because of block by intracellular Mg^{2+}. Native K_{ATP} channels show such weak rectification. The recently cloned subnit rcK_{ATP}-1 showed many of the properties of K_{ATP} channels when expressed in ***Xenopus*** oocytes, being inhibited by ATP, activated after run down by MgUDP, and activated by pinacidil (91). It was not, however, sensitive to sulphonylureas and a distinct sulphonylurea receptor has also been cloned recently (92). Krapivinsky et al (93) have also cloned an inward rectifier subunit, CIR (cardiac inward rectifier) that is essentially the same as rcK_{ATP}-1, differing in only two amino acids. In four expression systems CIR formed a K^+ channel, but the channel was not inhibited by ATP, nor opened by pinacidil. However, co-expression of CIR and GIRK1 forms a channel with properties identical to the native K_{ACh} of heart. Krapivinsky et al consider that the functional K_{ATP} channel protein complex is not yet resolved, but that it might consist of CIR combined with a different subunit or subunits to form a heteromultimer, perhaps including the sulphonylurea receptor.

REFERENCES

1. Nicholls CG, Lederer WJ. (1991) Adenosine triphosphate-sensitive potassium channels in the cardiovascular system. *Am. J. Physiol.* **261**:H1675-H1686.
2. Davies NW, Standen NB, Stanfield PR. (1991) ATP-dependent potassium channels of muscle cells: their properties, regulation and possible functions. *J. Bioenergetics Biomembr.* **23**, 509-535.
3. Noma A. (1993) Gating properties of ATP-sensitive K^+ channels in the heart. *Cardiovasc. Drugs Ther.* **7**, 515-520.
4. Takano M, Noma A. (1993) The ATP-sensitive K^+ channel. *Prog. Neurobiol.* **41**, 21-30.
5. Terzic A, Tung RT, Kurachi Y. (1994) Nucleotide regulation of ATP sensitive potassium channels. *Cardiovasc. Res.* **28**, 746-753.
6. Quayle JM, Standen NB. (1994) K_{ATP} channels in vascular smooth muscle. *Cardiovasc. Res.* **28**, 797-804.
7. Hille B. (1992) *Ionic Channels of Excitable Membranes.* Potassium channel pharmacology. Sunderland: Sinauer.
8. Escande D, Standen NB. (1993) eds. *K^+ Channels in Cardiovascular Medicine.* Paris: Springer-Verlag.
9. Noma A. (1983) ATP-regulated K^+ channels in cardiac muscle. *Nature.* **305**, 147-148.
10. Findlay I, Faivre J-F. (1991) ATP-sensitive K^+ channels in heart muscle. Spare channels. *FEBS Lett.* **279**, 95-97.

11. Lederer WJ, Nichols CG. (1989) Nucleotide modulation of the activity of rat heart ATP-sensitive K^+ channels in isolated membrane patches. *J. Physiol.* **419,** 193-211.

12. Davies NW, Standen NB, Stanfield PR. (1992) The effect of intracellular pH on ATP-dependent potassium channels of frog skeletal muscle. *J. Physiol.* **445,** 549-568.

13. Deutsch N, Matsuoka S, Weiss JN. (1994) Surface charge and properties of cardiac ATP-sensitive K^+ channels. *J. Gen. Physiol.* **104,** 773-800.

14. Elliot AC, Smith GL, Allen DG. (1994) Simultaneous measurement of action potential duration and intracellular ATP in isolated ferret hearts exposed to cyanide. *Circ. Res.* **64,** 583-591.

15. Weiss JN, Lamp ST. (1989) Cardiac ATP-sensitive K^+ channels. Evidence for preferential regulation by glycolysis. *J. Gen. Physiol.* **94,** 911-935.

16. Weiss JN, Venkatash N. (1993) Metabolic regulation of cardiac ATP-sensitive K^+ channels. *Cardiovasc. Drugs Ther.* **7,** 499-505.

17. Findlay I. (1988) Effects of ADP upon the ATP-sensitive K^+ channel in rat ventricular myocytes. *J. Membr. Biol.* **101,** 83-92.

18. Koyano T, Kakei M, Nakashima H, Yoshinaga M, Matsuoka T, Tanaka H. (1993) ATP-regulated K^+ channels are modulated by intracellular pH in guinea-pig ventricular cells. *J. Physiol.* **463,** 747-766.

19. Keung EC, Li Q. (1991) Lactate activates ATP-sensitive potassium channels in guinea-pig ventricular myocytes. *J. Clin. Invest.* **88,** 1772-1777.

20. Han J, So I, Kim EY, Earm YE. (1993) ATP-sensitive potassium channels are modulated by intracellular lactate in rabbit ventricular myocytes. *Pflügers Arch.* **425,** 546-548.

21. Kirsch GE, Codina J, Birnbaumer L, Brown AM. (1990) Coupling of ATP-sensitive K^+ channels to A_1 receptors by G proteins in rat ventricular myocytes. *Am. J. Physiol.* **259**, H820-H826.

22. Terzic A, Tung RT, Inanobe A, Katada T, Kurachi Y. (1994) G proteins activate ATP-sensitive K^+ channels by antagonizing ATP-dependent gating. *Neuron* **12,** 885-893.

23. Ito H, Vereecke J, Carmeliet E. (1994) Mode of regulation by G protein of the ATP-sensitive K^+ channel in guinea-pig ventricular cell membrane. *J. Physiol.* **478,** 101-108.

24. Ito H, Tung RT, Sugimoto T, Kobayashi I, Takahashi K, Katada T, Ui M, Kurachi Y. (1992) On the mechanism of G protein $\beta\gamma$ subunit activation of the muscarinic K^+ channel in guinea-pig atrial cell membrane. Comparison with the ATP-sensitive K^+ channel. *J. Gen. Physiol.* **99,** 961-983.

25. Dart C, Standen NB. (1993) Adenosine-activated potassium current in smooth muscle cells isolated from the pig coronary artery. *J. Physiol.* **471**, 767-786.

26. Quayle JM, Bonev AD, Brayden JE, Nelson MT. (1994) Calcitonin gene-related peptide activates ATP-sensitive K^+ currents in rabbit arterial smooth muscle via protein kinase A. *J. Physiol.* **475**, 9-13.

27. Miyoshi Y, Nakaya Y. (1991) Angiotensin II blocks ATP-sensitive K^+ channels in porcine coronary artery smooth muscle cells. *Biochem. Biophys. Res. Comm.* **181**, 700-706.

28. Miyoshi Y, Nakaya Y, Wakatsuki T, Nakaya S, Fujino K, Saito K, Inoue I. (1992) Endothelin blocks ATP-sensitive K^+ channels and depolarizes smooth muscle cells of porcine coronary artery. *Circ. Res.* **70**, 612-616.

29. Wakatsuki T, Nakaya Y, Inoue I. (1992) Vasopressin modulates K^+-channel activities of cultured smooth muscle cells from porcine coronary artery. *Am. J. Physiol.* **263**, H491-H496.

30. Bonev AD, Nelson MT. (1993) Muscarinic inhibition of ATP-sensitive K^+ channels by protein kinase C in urinary bladder smooth muscle. *Am. J. Physiol.* **265**, C1723-C1728.

31. Kakei M, Noma A, Shibasaki T. (1985) Properties of adenosine-triphosphate-regulated potassium channels in guinea-pig ventricular cells. *J. Physiol.* **363**, 441-462.

32. Takano M, Qin D, Noma A. (1990) ATP-dependent decay and recovery of K^+ channel in guinea-pig cardiac myocytes. *Am. J. Physiol.* **258**, H45-H50.

33. Findlay I. (1988) Calcium-dependent inactivation of the ATP-sensitive K^+ channel of rat ventricular myocytes. *Biochim. Biophys. Acta* **943**, 297-304.

34. Furukawa T, Fan Z, Sawanobori T, Hiraoka M. (1993) Modification of the ATP 5′-triphosphate-sensitive K^+ channel by trypsin in guinea-pig ventricular myocytes. *J. Physiol.* **466**, 707-726.

35. Furukawa T, Virag L, Furukawa N, Sawanobori T, Hiraoka M. (1994) Mechanism for reactivation of the ATP-sensitive K^+ channel by MgATP complexes in guinea-pig ventricular myocytes. *J. Physiol.* **479**, 95-107.

36. Tung RT, Kurachi Y. (1991) On the mechanism of nucleotide diphosphate activation of the ATP-sensitive K^+ channel in ventricular cell of guinea-pig. *J. Physiol.* **437**, 239-256.

37. Terzic A, Findlay I, Hosoya Y, Kurachi Y. (1994) Dualistic behavior of the ATP-sensitive K^+ channel toward intracellular nucleoside diphosphates. *Neuron* **12**, 1049-1058.

38. Kajioka S, Kitamura K, Kuriyama H. (1991) Guanosine diphosphate activates an adenosine-5'-triphosphate-sensitive K^+ channel in the rabbit portal vein. *J. Physiol.* **444**, 397-418.

39. Beech DJ, Zhang H, Nakao K, Bolton TB. (1993) K channel activation by nucleotide diphosphates and its inhibition by glibenclamide in vascular smooth muscle cells. *Br. J. Pharmacol.* **110**, 573-582.

40. Zhang H, Bolton TB. (1995) Activation by intracellular GDP, metabolic inhibition and pinacidil of a glibenclamide-sensitive K-channel in smooth muscle cells of rat mesenteric artery. *Br. J. Pharmacol.* **114**, 662-672.

41. Cook NS, Quast U. (1990) Potassium channel pharmacology. In *Potassium Channels. Structure, Classification, Function and Therapeutic Potential*, ed. Cook, N.S., pp. 181-255. Chichester: Ellis Horwood.

42. Edwards G, Weston AH. (1993) The pharmacology of ATP-sensitive K channels. *Ann. Rev. Pharmacol. Toxicol.* **33**, 597-637.

43. Fosset M, De Weille JR, Green RD, Schmid-Antomarchi H, Lazdunski M. (1988) Antidiabetic sulfonylureas control action potential properties in heart cells via high affinity receptors that are linked to ATP-dependent K^+ channels. *J. Biol. Chem.* **263**, 7933-7936.

44. Escande D, Thuringer D, Le Guern s, Courteix J, Laville M, Cavero I. (1989) Potassium channel openers act through an activation of ATP-sensitive K^+ channels in guinea-pig cardiac myocytes. *Pflügers Arch.* **414**, 669-675.

45. Findlay I. (1992) Inhibition of ATP-sensitive K^+ channels in cardiac muscle by the sulphonylurea drug glibenclamide. *J. Pharmacol. Exp. Ther.* **261**, 540-545.

46. Findlay I. (1993) Sulphonylurea drugs no longer inhibit ATP-sensitive K^+ channels during metabolic stress in cardiac muscle. *J. Pharmacol. Exp. Ther.* **266**, 456-467.

47. Cavero I, Guillon JM. (1993) Pharmacological profile of potassium channel openers in the vasculature. In *K^+ Channels in Cardiovascular Medicine*. ed. Escande D, Standen NB. pp. 193-223. Paris: Springer-Verlag.

48. Escande D, Cavero I. (1993) Potassium channel openers in the heart. In *K^+ Channels in Cardiovascular Medicine*. ed. Escande D, Standen NB. pp. 193-223. Paris: Springer-Verlag.

49. Henry P, Escande D. (1994) Do potassium channel openers compete with ATP to activate ATP sensitive potassium channels? *Cardiovasc. Res.* **28**, 754-759.

50. Thuringer D, Escande D. (1994) Apparent competition between ATP and the potassium channel opener RP49356 on ATP-sensitive K^+ channels of cardiac myocytes. *Mol. Pharmacol.* **36**, 897-902.

51. Gasser RNA, Vaughan-Jones RD. (1990) Mechanism of potassium efflux and action potential shortening during ischaemia in isolated mammalian cardiac muscle. *J. Physiol.* **431,** 713-741.
52. Wilde AAM, Escande D, Schumacher CA, Thuringer D, Mestre M, Fiolet JWT, Janse MJ. (1990) Potassium accumulation in globally ischaemic mammalian heart: A role for the ATP-sensitive potassium channel. *Circ. Res.* **67,** 835-843.
53. Cole WC, McPherson CD, Sonntag D. (1991) ATP-regulated K^+ channels protect the myocardium against ischaemia/reperfusion damage. *Circ. Res.* **69,** 571-581.
54. Weiss JN, Venkatesh N, Lamp ST. (1992) ATP-sensitive K^+ channels and cellular K^+ loss in hypoxic and ischaemic mammalian ventricle. *J. Physiol.* **447,** 649-673.
55. Notsu T, Tanaka I, Takano M, Noma A. (1993) Blockade of the ATP-sensitive K^+ channel by 5-hydroxdecanoate in guinea pig ventricular myocytes. *Circ. Res.* **72,** 560-570.
56. Billman GE (1994) Role of ATP sensitive potassium channel in extracellular potassium accumulation and cardiac arrhythmias during myocardial ischaemia. *Cardiovasc. Res.* **28,** 762-769.
57. Lederer WJ, Nichols CG, Smith GL. (1991) The mechanism of early contractile failure of isolated rat ventricular myocytes subjected to complete metabolic inhibition. *J. Physiol.* **413,** 329-349.
58. Vanheel B, de Hemptinne A. (1992) Influence of K_{ATP} channel on modulation of net potassium efflux from ischaemic mammalian cardiac tissue. *Cardiovasc. Res.* **26,** 1030-1039.
59. Mitani A, Kinoshita K, Fukamachi K, Sakamoto M, Kurisu K, Tsuruhara Y, Fukumura F, Nakashima A, Tokunaga K. (1991) Effects of glibenclamide and nicorandil on cardiac function during ischaemia and reperfusion in isolated perfused rat hearts. *Am. J. Physiol.* **261,** H1864-H1871.
60. Nelson MT, Patlak JB, Worley JF, Standen NB. (1990) Calcium channels, potassium channels, and voltage-dependence of arterial smooth muscle tone. *Am. J. Physiol.* **259,** C3-C18.
61. Hirst GDS, Edwards FR. (1989) Sympathetic neuroeffector transmission in arteries and arterioles. *Physiol. Rev.* **69,** 546-604.
62. Itoh T, Seki N, Suzuki S, Ito S, Kajikura J, Kuriyama H. (1992) Membrane hyperpolarization inhibits agonist-induced synthesis of inositol 1,4,5,-trisphosphate in rabbit mesenteric artery. *J. Physiol.* **451,** 307-328.

63. Ganitkevich VY, Isenberg G. (1993) Membrane potential modulates inositol 1,4,5-trisphosphate-mediated Ca^{2+} transients in guinea pig coronary myocytes. *J. Physiol.* **470**, 35-44.

64. Daut J, Maier-Rudolph W, von Beckerath N, Mehrke G, Gunther K, Goedel-Meinen L. (1990) Hypoxic vasodilation of coronary arteries is mediated by ATP-sensitive potassium channels. *Science* **247**:1341-1344.

65. Jackson WF. (1993) Arteriolar tone is determined by activity of ATP-sensitive potassium channels. *Am. J. Physiol.* **265**, H1797-H1803.

66. Nakhostine N, Lamontagne D. (1993) Adenosine contributes to hypoxia-induced vasodilation through ATP-sensitive K^+ channel activation. *Am. J. Physiol.* **265**, H1289-H1293.

67. Marshall JM, Thomas T, Turner L. (1993) A link between adenosine, ATP-sensitive K^+ channels, potassium and muscle vasodilation in the rat in systemic hypoxia. *J. Physiol.* **472**, 1-9.

68. Reid JM, Paterson DJ, Ashcroft FM, Bergel DH. The effect of tolbutamide on cerebral blood flow during hypoxia and hypercapnia in the anaesthetized rat. *Pflügers Arch.* 1993; **425**, 362-364.

69. Dart C, Standen NB. (1995) Activation of ATP-dependent K^+ channels by hypoxia in smooth muscle cells isolated from the pig coronary artery. *J. Physiol.* **483**, 29-39.

70. von Beckerath N, Cyrys S, Dischner A, Daut J. (1991) Hypoxic vasodilatation in isolated, perfused guinea-pig heart: an analysis of the underlying mechanisms. *J. Physiol.* **442**, 297-319.

71. Park KH, Rubin LE, Gross SS, Levi R. (1992) Nitric oxide is a mediator of hypoxic coronary vasodilation: Relation to adenosine and cyclooxygenase-derived metabolites. *Circ. Res.* **71**, 992-1001.

72. Narisige T, Egashira K, Akatsuka Y, Katsuda Y, Numaguchi K, Sakata M, Takeshita A. (1993) Glibenclamide, a putative ATP-sensitive K^+ channel blocker, inhibits coronary autoregulation in anaesthetized dogs. *Circ. Res.* **73**, 771-776.

73. Komaru T, Lamping KG, Eastham CL, Dellsperger KC. (1991) Role of ATP-sensitive potassium channels in coronary microvascular autoregulatory responses. *Circ. Res.* **69**, 1146-1151.

74. Hong KW, Pyo KM, Lee WS, Yu SS, Rhim BY. (1994) Pharmacological evidence that calcitonin gene-related peptide is implicated in cerebral autoregulation. *Am. J. Physiol.* **266**, H11-H16.

75. Samaha FF, Heineman FW, Ince C, Fleming J, Balaban RS. (1992) ATP-sensitive potassium channel is essential to maintain basal coronary vascular tone *in vivo*. *Am. J. Physiol.* **262**, C1220-C1227.
76. Duncker DJ, Van Zon NS, Altman JD, Pavek, TJ, Bache RJ. (1993) Role of K^{+}_{ATP} channels in coronary vasodilation during exercise. *Circ. Res.* **88**, 1245-1253.
77. Eckman DM, Frankovich JD, Keef KD. (1992) Comparison of the actions of acetylcholine and BRL 38227 in the guinea pig coronary artery. *Br. J. Pharmacol.* **106**, 9-16.
78. McPherson GA, Angus JA. (1991) Evidence that acetylcholine-mediated hyperpolarization of the rat small mesenteric artery does not involve the K^+ channel opened by cromakalim. *Br. J. Pharmacol.* **103**, 1184-1190.
79. Clapp LH, Gurney AM. (1992) ATP-sensitive K^+ channels regulate resting potential of pulmonary arterial smooth muscle cells. *Am. J. Physiol.* **262**, H916-H920.
80. Nelson MT, Huang Y, Brayden JE, Hescheler J, Standen NB. (1990) Arterial dilations in response to calcitonin gene-related peptide involve activation of K^+ channels. *Nature* **344**, 70-773.
81. Standen NB, Quayle JM, Davies NW, Brayden JE, Huang Y, Nelson MT. (1989) Hyperpolarizing vasodilators activate ATP-sensitive K^+ channels in arterial smooth muscle. *Science* **245**, 177-180.
82. Brayden JE. (1990) Membrane hyperpolarisation is a mechanism of endothelium-dependent cerebral vasodilation. *Am. J. Physiol.* **259**, H668-H673.
83. Brayden JE. (1993) Hyperpolarization and relaxation of resistance arteries in response to adenosine diphosphate. *Circ. Res.* **69**, 1415-1420.
84. Kubo M, Nakaya Y, Matsuoka S, Saito K, Kuroda Y. (1994) Atrial natriuretic factor and isosorbide dinitrate modulate the gating of ATP-sensitive K^+ channels in cultured vascular smooth muscle cells. *Circ. Res.* **74**, 471-476.
85. Quayle JM, McCarron JG, Brayden JE, Nelson MT. (1993) Inward rectifier K^+ currents in smooth muscle cells from rat resistance-sized cerebral arteries. *Am. J. Physiol.* **264**, C1363-C1370.
86. Horie M, Irisawa H, Noma A. (1987) Voltage-dependent magnesium block of adenosine-triphosphate-sensitive potassium channel in guinea-pig ventricular cells. *J. Physiol.* **387**, 251-272.
87. Jan LY, Jan YN. (1992) Structural elements involved in specific K^+ channel functions. *Ann. Rev. Physiol.* **54**, 537-555.

88. Kubo Y, Baldwin TJ, Jan YN, Yan LY. (1993) Primary structure and functional expression of a mouse inward rectifier potassium channel. *Nature* **362**, 127-133.

89. Lopatin A, Makhina EN, Nichols CG. (1994) Potassium channel block by cytoplasmic polyamines as the mechanism of intrinsic rectification. *Nature* **372**, 366-369.

90. Fakler B, Brändle U, Glowatzki E, Weidemann S, Zenner H-P, Ruppersberg JP. (1995) Strong voltage-dependent inward rectification of inward rectifier K^+ channels is caused by intracellular spermine. *Cell* **80**, 149-154.

91. Ashford MLJ, Bond CT, Blair, Adelman JP. (1994) Cloning and functional expression of a rat heart K_{ATP} channel. *Nature* **370**, 456-459.

92. Aguilar-Bryan L, Clememt J, Nelson DA, Bryan J. (1995) Expression and characterization of a cloned high affinity sulphonylurea receptor. *Biophys. J.* **68**, A234.

93. Krapivinsky G, Gordon EA, Wickman K, Velimirovic B, Krapivinsky L, Clapham DE. (1995) The G-protein-gated atrial K^+ channel I_{KACh} is a heteromultimer of two inwardly rectifying K^+-channel proteins. *Nature* **374**, 135-141.

2

VASCULAR PATHOLOGY AND THE K_{ATP} CHANNEL

ULRICH QUAST and STEFAN GLOCKER

Department of Pharmacology, Medical Faculty, University of Tübingen, Wilhelmstr. 56, D-72074 Tübingen, Germany.

INTRODUCTION

K^+ channels determine the resting membrane potential and cellular excitability of most cells [1]. The opening of K^+ channels shifts the membrane potential towards the K^+ equilibrium potential which is around -90 mV. In excitable cells endowed with depolarization-activated Ca^{2+} channels (voltage-gated Ca^{2+} channels, VOCCs), hyperpolarization will prevent such channels from opening and block Ca^{2+} entry via this pathway. In cells devoid of VOCCs or in cells where these channels are not important for Ca^{2+} entry, e.g. endothelial cells, leukocytes and others, hyper-polarization will increase the driving force for Ca^{2+} entry into the cell and promote Ca^{2+} influx into the cell via pathways which are active at such hyperpolarized membrane potentials [2]. In this article we will shortly review the major classes of K^+ channels and consider their physiological role in vascular smooth muscle cells, endothelial cells and macrophages. Emphasis will be placed on vascular ATP-sensitive K^+ channels (K_{ATP} channels) and their modulaton in normal and pathological states.

MAJOR CLASSES OF K^+ CHANNELS

Most K^+ channels known to date show a fourfold symmetry, their pore forming (α-) subunits being assembled in form of a tetramer [1,3]; this basic unit is often complemented by additional subunits (termed β-, γ-, δ- etc subunits) which are important for modulation of channel activity. There are two different types of K^+ channel α-subunits which are characterized by the number of α-helical segments spanning the membrane and which determine whether the channel falls into the superfamily of the voltage-gated or the inwardly rectifying K^+ channels (K_{IR}) (Fig. 1). α-subunits of K_{IR} channels contain two transmembrane segments (M1 and M2) which are linked by an extracellular loop (H5); this loop folds back into the membrane and contributes to the lining of the channel pore (Fig. 1). The cardiac K_{ATP} channel appears to belong to this superfamily (see below). α-subunits of voltage-gated K^+ channels have 6 transmembrane segments designated S1 to S6 with the H5 loop connecting S5 and S6 ([1,3], Fig. 1); the S4 segment consists of four to five motifs where two hydrophobic amino acids are followed by a positively charged one generating a strong dipole moment in the membrane. Therefore, the S4 segment is supposed to constitute the voltage sensor of the channel which triggers the conformational changes leading to channel opening upon depolarization [1,3]. The S4 segment may have additional (structural) functions and, in some cases, it confers only a weak voltage dependence to the channel which is gated by other mechanisms like e.g. cyclic nucleotide binding (cyclic nucleotide-gated cation channel) [4].

Voltage-dependent K^+ channels

Functionally, voltage-gated K^+ channels fall into two broad categories, i.e. channels which open rapidly in response to depolarization and inactivate quite rapidly again if depolarization is sustained (A channels, K_A), and channels which may open more slowly and inactivate much more slowly (delayed rectifier K^+ channels, K_V); some of these K_V channels do not inactivate at all over many minutes [1,3].

Channel	γ (pS)	I-V Curve	Pharmacology	Folding
K_V	~15	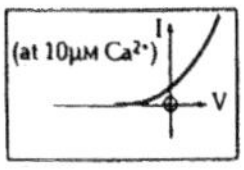	B: sotalol dofetilide E 4031	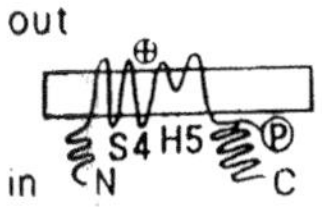
BK_{Ca}	150	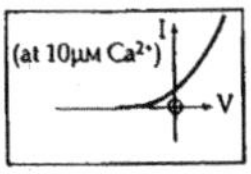	B: CTX, ITX O: saponins NS 1619	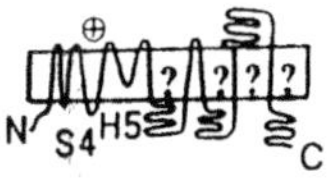
K_{IR}	15	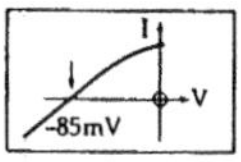	B: terikalant	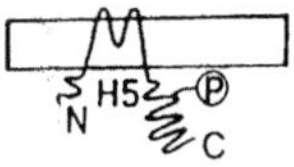
K_{ATP}	15	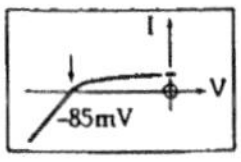	B: sulphonylureas O: levcromakalim P1075 aprikalim	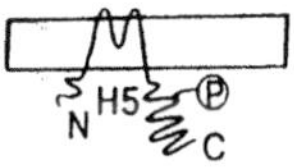

Fig. 1: Properties of major K^+ channels. The abbreviations denoting the channels are those used in the text; The values appearing under γ give the single channel conductance in pS under quasiphysiological conditions. The formulae of the channel modulators (O = opener, B = blocker) listed under 'pharmacology' are compiled in ref. [8]. The last column shows the (putative) folding of the α-subunit of the channel.

Both groups of channels let the K^+ current pass only out of the cell (outward rectifiers) and they are both of great importance for repolarization of the cell; in addition, K_A channels are involved in setting the firing frequency of pacemaker cells [1]. Blockers of cardiac K_V channels prolong the action potential and are in development as class III anti-arrhythmic agents [5]. In human T lymphocytes, block of the K_V channel ($K_V1.3$) depolarizes the cell, inhibits Ca^{2+} entry and prevents the subsequent lymphokine production by and the proliferation of these cells. Hence, selective blockers of this channel in lymphocytes may be novel immunosuppressant agents [6].

Detailed investigations have elucidated the domains which are responsible for the voltage dependence (S4 segment), which make up the pore (H5 loop and parts of S6 segment and the S4-S5 loop), which determine the pharmacological properties and which govern the rapid inactivation of some K_V channels according to a ball and chain model [3,7]. Very recently, a cytosolic protein has been cloned which associates in a 1:1 stoichiometry with the α-subunits of the K_V1 channel to form a $\alpha_4\beta_4$ heterotetrameric complex [7]. Interestingly, the channel formed by the α-subunits alone shows very slow inactivation; association with the ß-subunits confers the rapid (A-type) inactivation to this channel, an effect mediated by a domain in the amino terminus of the ß-subunit which acts as the inactivation ball [7].

Ca-dependent K^+ channels (K_{Ca})

Ca^{2+}-sensitive K^+ channels (K_{Ca} channels) have the important function to couple the membrane potential to the intracellular Ca^{2+} concentration [1]. According to their unitary conductance, K_{Ca} channels are divided into three heterogeneous groups with small, intermediate and large ("big") conductance, respectively (SK_{Ca}, IK_{CA} and BK_{Ca} channels; [1,8,9]). Here we focus on BK_{Ca} channels; these have a conductance of 100 - 200 pS under quasi-physiological conditions and form a heterogeneous and almost ubiquitous class of K^+ channels. They open at depolarized membrane potentials in response to elevated intracellular Ca^{2+} concentrations [1,8]. Recently, BK_{Ca} channel α-subunits have been cloned from *Drosophila* and from murine skeletal muscle [10-12]; the amino-terminal part of the protein is homologous to the α-subunit of voltage-gated (K_A and K_V) K^+ channels; this is followed by a very long C-terminal part with unknown structure (Fig. 1). The native channel in smooth muscle also comprises a β-subunit with two putative transmembrane segments [13].

In addition to the gating of the BK_{Ca} channels by depolarization and elevated intracellular Ca^{2+} their activity in some tissues is modulated by cAMP-dependent phosphorylation, G-proteins, the guanine nucleotides GMP and cGMP and other factors (reviewed in [8,9]). Toxins like charybdotoxin and iberiotoxin and non-peptidyl indole diterpenes like paxilline block BK_{Ca} channels with high affinity (references in [14]). Recently, a chemically heterogeneous group of compounds has been discovered which activate the channel. These BK_{Ca} openers are potentially of great therapeutic interest [8,14].

The superfamily of inwardly rectifying K^+ channels (K_{IR})

K_{IR} channels are characterized by the property of conducting K^+ more efficiently into the cell than in the outward direction [1]. They are activated by hyperpolarization (e.g when membrane potential is more negative than the K^+ equilibrium potential); in many cells they determine the resting membrane potential [1]. K_{IR} channels (more precisely their α-subunits) have been cloned recently from several sources ([15], further references in [3]); their putative folding is shown in Fig. 1. The degree of rectification varies amongst different members of the K_{IR} channel family as do the intrinsic voltage dependence and the kinetics of opening. These differences are now explained in terms of differences in the voltage-dependent block of these channels by Mg^{2+} (references in [3]) and polyamines like spermine [16]. The molecular basis for these differences is being unravelled now by site directed mutagenesis and the construction of chimeras; these studies point at the importance of the negatively charged amino acid Asp at position 172 in the M2 segment and of the hydrophylic (intracellular) C-terminal domain [3]. Recent cloning results have revealed that the muscarinic receptor regulated K^+ channel in rat atrium (cloned α-subunit GIRK1, [17]) and the K_{ATP} channel (cloned variant rcK_{ATP}-1 ([18], see also [67]) both belong to the K_{IR} channel superfamily. GIRK1 is directly activated by the βγ-subunits of the G-protein, G_i [19] and mediates the decrease in cardiac frequency following cholinergic stimulation. Regulation of K^+ channels by G-proteins and thus by neurotransmitters and hormones constitutes a very important signalling pathway [20]. It seems noteworthy that in the heart the α-subunit of G_i activates the K_{ATP} channel whereas the βγ-subunits stimulate GIRK1 [21].

ATP-sensitive K^+ channels (K_{ATP} channels)

K_{ATP} channels are closed by ATP binding to an intracellular binding site; they open when ATP dissociates from this site and/or when Mg^{2+} salts of nucleoside diphosphates (NDP) like MgADP and MgGDP bind to an activatory site which is different from the inhibitory ATP site. Thus, the opening of K_{ATP} channels is regulated by the quotient of ATP/NDP; hence, these channels link cellular excitability to the metabolic state of the cell [8, 22-24]. The K_{ATP} channels constitute a heterogeneous class of K^+ channels found in excitable tissues like heart, skeletal and smooth muscle, neurons, pancreatic ß-cells [22,23] and the rat adenohypophysis, but also in tissues like kidney epithelium or the follicular cells surrounding the Xenopus oocyte (for references see [24]). As with many other ion channels, the activity of K_{ATP} channels is also modulated by phosphorylation [8,22-24]. A characteristic feature of K_{ATP} channels is their inhibition by sulphonylureas like glibenclamide with widely varying affinities in different tissues [8,22-26]. In many tissues, the K_{ATP} channels are opened by a structurally heterogeneous class of compounds, the K_{ATP} channel openers, which include nicorandil (an agent which also acts as a nitrate, increasing cGMP), minoxidil sulphate, pinacidil, diazoxide, cromakalim and aprikalim [8,23,25].

Under quasiphysiological conditions, K_{ATP} channels exhibit single channel conductances between 15 to 40 pS and, in general, a slight inward rectification [8,22]. Interestingly, the recently cloned rcK_{ATP}-1 channel showed, after heterologous expression in a kidney epithelial cell line, many of the hallmarks of a typical K_{ATP} channel [18]; however, the most recent data suggest that the native K_{ATP} channel may be a heteromultimer of four K_{IR} α-subunits perhaps including the sulphonylurea receptor as regulator [27]. Indeed, rcK_{ATP}-1 was insensitive to inhibition by glibenclamide [18], demonstrating that the sulphonylurea binding site is not part of the cloned channel. Two high affinity sulphonylurea binding proteins have been purified: one of them is a 38 kD protein [28]; the other, a 140 kD protein, has recently been cloned from a ß-cell line and shown to belong to the ABC (ATP Binding Cassette) protein superfamily; however, this protein appears to have 13 transmembrane segments instead of 12 as is usual with ABC proteins [29].

The physiological role of K_{ATP} channels depends on the tissue. In the pancreatic ß-cell, K_{ATP} channels determine the resting membrane potential and regulate insulin release in response to the plasma glucose level. Plasma glucose, when taken up by the the ß-cell, leads to an increase in the ATP concentration near the channel. Subsequent closing of the K_{ATP} channel depolarizes the ß-cell and leads to Ca^{2+} entry into the cell via VOCCs, thus inducing insulin secretion. The sulphonylureas are blockers optimized for this channel in the ß-cell and are still of major importance in the treatment of non-insulin-dependent diabetes [22]. In many tissues, however, K_{ATP} channels are closed under physiological conditions; they open when the tissue is metabolically compromised, i.e. the quotient of ATP/NDP falls. Their opening clamps the cell in the resting state thus saving ATP and helping the cell to survive [30]. The fact that the K_{ATP} channel openers act on precisely the K^+ channel that opens under ischemic and hypoxic conditions may explain the therapeutic benefit found with these compounds in animal models of cardioprotection ([30], see also chapters by Hearse and Gross & Yellon) and intermittent claudication [31].

K^+ CHANNELS IN MACROPHAGES AND VASCULAR TISSUE

In the pathogenesis of vascular diseases the interactions between vascular smooth muscle, the endothelium and cells of the inflammatory and immune system are of major importance. In the following we will shortly review the major K^+ channels found in macrophages, the prototype cells of the inflammatory system, in endothelial and in vascular smooth muscle cells with particular emphasis on K_{ATP} channels.

K^+ channels in macrophages

Macrophages, like lymphocytes, belong to the class of 'non-excitable cells' where dihydropyridine-sensitive Ca^{2+}channels (VOCCs) are absent (or do not contribute to any significant degree to Ca^{2+} entry) [32,2]. It is important for development of the full biological response after stimulation that these cells do not depolarize since depolarization of macrophages (e.g. by block of K^+ channels or by high KCl) inhibits cytokine secretion [33], probably by reducing the driving force for Ca^{2+} entry into the cell [2]. The major K^+ conductances fall into three classes, inwardly rectifying, outwardly conducting and Ca^{2+}-dependent. An inward rectifier has recently been cloned from mouse macrophages; it belongs to the group of strong rectifiers [34]. In agreement with the properties of the macroscopic inward conductance [32] the presumed role of this channel is to contribute to the resting potential of the cell as its block by Ba^{2+} at mM concentrations depolarizes the cell. Two outwardly rectifying conductances have been identified, one inactivating and one non-inactivating. The latter resembles very much the outward rectifying conductance in lymphocytes [32], where the *Shaker* type $K_V1.3$ channel has been shown to underlie this current. This channel is probably important in opposing major depolarizations of the macrophage once the membrane potential stabilizing effect of the K_{IR} channel has been overrun. In T lymphocytes, however, the $K_V1.3$ channel sets the resting membrane potential [6]. The BK_{Ca} channel is the major Ca^{2+}-dependent K^+ conductance in the macrophage; it too opposes or terminates large depolarizations [32]. The current-voltage relationship of macrophages is N-shaped and flat, compatible with a bimodal distribution of the resting membrane potential around values of -70 and -15 mV.

K^+ channels in the endothelium

The endothelium functions not only as a barrier of varying permeability between blood and vascular smooth muscle, it also contributes to the regulation of vascular tone primarily by the secretion of vasoactive substances like endothelium-derived relaxing factor (EDRF = NO), endothelin and others [35,36]; in addition it secretes many factors important in haemostasis (e.g. von Willebrand factor, PAI, TPA etc.) and angiogenesis (various mitogens and growth factors) [36]. Detailed investigations of the stimulus-secretion coupling in these cells have shown that, in general, an increase in intracellular Ca^{2+} is necessary for secretion; this Ca^{2+} increase is caused by mobilization from stores via the IP_3 signalling chain and by Ca^{2+} entry via several pathways, none of them being sensitive to inhibition by dihydropyridines [36-38]. Ca^{2+} entry into endothelial cells generally requires a maintained polarization [37,39,40].

Major K^+ conductances in endothelial cells are K_{IR}, K_V, K_A, BK_{Ca} and an inwardly rectifying K^+ channel activated by shear stress (reviews [37,38]). Similar to the findings with macrophages the current-voltage relationship of endothelial cells is determined by the contributions from K_{IR} and K_V resulting in a flat N-shaped curve. This allows again a bimodal distribution of the resting membrane potential around values of -80 and -25 mV [40]; the actual value may depend on culture conditions and on the vascular origin of the cells [37,38]. The BK_{Ca} channels may contribute to the hyperpolarization following application of Ca^{2+} mobilizing hormones which augments the driving force for Ca^{2+} entry into the cell [38,40]. The resulting Ca^{2+} transient stimulates EDRF (NO) generation by activating NO synthase which is, in its constitutive form, a Ca^{2+}/calmodulin-dependent enzyme [37]. NO diffuses freely out of the cell and stimulates the production of cGMP in smooth muscle cells and platelets, thereby reducing vascular tone and platelet activity.

Evidence of the occurrence of K_{ATP} channels in endothelial cells has been obtained directly [41] or indirectly [39], but has not been found by others [40]. In any event, it has been generally found that the effects of the K_{ATP} channel openers on vascular smooth muscle are independent of the presence of the endothelium (but see effects of openers on dog coronary artery *in vivo* [42]).

K^+ channels in vascular smooth muscle

K^+ channels of major importance in vascular smooth muscle include K_v, K_A, BK_{Ca}, K_{ATP} and K_{IR} channels [8,43-45]. K_{IR} channels have been found in arterioles [46,47] where they are, together with BK_{Ca} channels, important contributors to the resting membrane potential which is around -50 mV. In larger vessels, however, K_{IR} seem to be absent [43,44,47] and it remains unclear which K^+ channels contribute to the the resting membrane potential there [44]; probably this depends on the nature of the vessel. K_V channels are important for repolarisation as are BK_{Ca} channels [43-45]. Due to their very large unitary conductance, the opening of a few BK_{Ca} channels will have a great impact on membrane potential. The recently described BK_{Ca} channel openers are obviously of greatest interest [14,8]; however, the compounds available still suffer from various problems like lack of specificity, lack of cell penetration and others [14,24,43]. The role of the K_A channel is unclear in quiescent vessels; in spontanously active vessels like the rat portal vein where an interburst membrane potential of -60 mV is reached, they may contribute to the resting membrane potential and affect pacemaker frequency [44].

Vascular K_{ATP} channels

The physiological role of K_{ATP} channels in vascular smooth muscle is not yet clear as the MgNDP/ATP ratio in vascular myocytes under normal conditions keeps the channel in the closed state. However, in some vascular beds these channels are opened by vasorelaxant neurotransmitters and hormones, probably via activation of a G-protein, thereby relaxing the vessel. Opening of K_{ATP} channels mediates the relaxation of the coronary vasculature by adenosine [48,49], prostacyclin or its analogue iloprost [50] and of mesenteric arterioles by calcitonin gene related peptide [51], whereas the contribution of K_{ATP} channel opening to the vasorelaxant effect of the endothelium-derived hyperpolarizing factor(s) (EDHF) seems to remain controversial (references in [8]). There is convincing evidence to show that the channel is also opened by depletion of intracellular ATP and/or an increase in MgNDP [52-55].

Vascular effects of the K_{ATP} channel openers

Channel opening: The most direct manifestation of the K_{ATP} channel openers is the induction of a K^+ current with biophysical and pharmacological properties which indicate that it is indeed flowing through the K_{ATP} channel described above. This current is directed outward, leading to hyperpolarization of the cell; it can also be monitored in tracer efflux experiments using $^{42}K^+$ or $^{86}Rb^+$as tracer ions (reviews [8,25]). The mechanism by which the K_{ATP} channel openers activate the channel in vascular smooth muscle is still a matter of debate [8,25]. Binding assays in rings of rat aorta using the tritiated pinacidil analogue, ^{3}H-P1075, suggest that the major K_{ATP} channel openers bind to the same target, but possibly to different sites at this target, to elicit their effects [56,57]. The sulphonylurea glibenclamide binds to a site different from and negatively allosterically coupled to the ^{3}H-P1075 binding site [56]. The question whether or not the drug receptor of the channel openers is the K_{ATP} channel itself or a protein different from it, must remain open at present since the biochemical characterization of the drug receptor for the openers is still lacking. The fact that K_{ATP} channel openers are able to open K_{ATP} channels in isolated patches from vascular smooth muscle cells (references in [8]) does not necessarily imply a direct action of these compounds on the channel since the isolated patch may contain proteins other than the α-subunits important for channel modulation.

Smooth muscle relaxation: The hyperpolarization of smooth muscle leads to relaxation and the K_{ATP} channel openers have been instrumental in the study of the relationship between membrane potential and the excitability of smooth muscle [58]. First, hyperpolarization clamps the cell at sufficiently negative values to prevent depolarization-induced Ca^{2+} entry by voltage-sensitive Ca^{2+} channels [59]; in this respect the openers may be looked at as indirect Ca^{2+} channel blockers. In addition, the K_{ATP} channel openers, by their hyperpolarizing action, inhibit the agonist-induced accumulation of IP_3, thus interfering with agonist-stimulated Ca^{2+} mobilization from intracellular stores; they also reduce the intracellular Ca^{2+} concentration in vascular smooth muscle at rest in both Ca^{2+}-containing and Ca^{2+}-free media and decrease the Ca^{2+}-sensitivity of the contractile elements in strips of canine coronary artery (references in [58]). The precise mechanism by which hyperpolarization of the cell membrane regulates these phenomena remains to be established. These actions of the K_{ATP} channel openers suggest that the smooth muscle relaxant profile of these compounds will differ from that of the Ca^{2+} antagonists and they explain earlier findings that the openers relax contractions which do not depend on depolarization-induced Ca^{2+} entry (references in [58]).

An additional complexity arises from experiments with the K^+ channel blockers tedisamil, Ba^{2+} and Rb^+. These studies show that the large majority of the K^+ channels opened by the openers can be blocked without much effect on smooth muscle relaxation. This suggests that these compounds possess mechanisms of vasorelaxation, independent of plasmalemmal K_{ATP} channel opening. One such mechanism is the (partial) inhibition of intracellular Ca^{2+} store refilling, produced by (lev)-cromakalim in vascular tissues (references in [58]).

The vasorelaxant effect of the K_{ATP} channel shows two characteristic traits: First, it is abolished in media containing high concentrations of K^+ [59] and second, it is inhibited by the sulphonylureas, in particular by glibenclamide [60]. It is important to note that glibenclamide inhibits both the K^+ channel opening and the vasorelaxant effects of the K_{ATP} channel openers at similar concentrations [60]. This implies that the 'additional' mechanisms of vasorelaxation (which are independent of plasmalemmal K_{ATP} channel opening) are also sensitive to depolarization and to inhibition by glibenclamide.

The antagonism by glibenclamide of the vasorelaxant and channel opening effects of the K_{ATP} openers often displays a competitive appearance (see e.g. [60]); however, as mentioned above, kinetic studies have shown that the openers and glibenclamide are not strictily competitive with one another but that they bind to two different sites which are negatively allosterically coupled [56]. In vascular smooth muscle, concentrations $\geq$ 100 nM are required to produce substantial inhibition of the vasorelaxant and $^{86}Rb^{+}$ efflux stimulating effects of the K_{ATP} channel openers (see e.g. [60]). At these concentration, however, but even more so in the μM range, glibenclamide has numerous additional effects unrelated to K_{ATP} channel blockade (references in [61]).

VASCULAR K_{ATP} CHANNELS IN PATHOLOGICAL CONDITIONS

Vascular effects of K_{ATP} channels openers in tissue ischemia

Skeletal muscle: In several animal species K_{ATP} channel openers produce only minor increases in skeletal muscle blood flow whereas Ca^{2+} antagonists prominently increase blood flow in this vascular bed (references in [31]). This profile is reversed in hypoxic skeletal muscle. In rat hindlimbs after formation of collaterals and induction of acute ischemia the K_{ATP} channel openers cromakalim, pinacidil and nicorandil (but not the calcium antagonists nor hydralazine) selectively increase blood cell flux and oxygen tension in the ischemic area [62]. In addition, the K_{ATP} channel openers accelerate the recovery of high energy phosphates after a period of transient ischemia at doses below those that lower blood pressure [31]. Recent studies in the isolated rabbit ear have shown that levcromakalim (but not verapamil or sodium nitroprusside) selectively improve collateral perfusion following arterial occlusion ([63] and references therein). These observations suggest that the K_{ATP} channel openers (at low doses) may be of therapeutic benefit in intermittent claudication, a situation with a great need for an improved pharmaceutical treatment.

Angina pectoris: The usefulness of a vasodilator in this indication depends on the ability to improve perfusion of the ischemic area. In order to avoid steal phenomena it seems important to dilate the large coronary arteries with atherosclerotic lesions more than resistance vessels; in addition, the vasodilator should not induce reflex tachycardia. The K_{ATP} channel openers are known to act preferentially on small arterioles and increase heart rate in response to blood pressure lowering in normotensive and hypertensive animals [64]. In addition, high doses of the openers induce a redistribution of blood flow from inner to outer layers of the rabbit heart [65] which may lead to subendocardial necroses upon prolonged treatment. Indeed, minoxidil is known for its propensity to aggravate ischemic symptoms in susceptible patients even after topical application at the skull to improve hair growth [66]. The possibility that the vasodilator effect of cromakalim and pinacidil in large coronary arteries depends on an intact endothelium [42] casts further doubt on the value of the K_{ATP} channel openers in the treatment of angina pectoris. On the other hand, it has been shown that the hypoxic dilation of coronary arteries is mediated by the opening of K_{ATP} channels [48]. This may be mediated, at least in part, via the release of adenosine which opens K_{ATP} in the coronary artery [48,49] so that the K_{ATP} channel openers may exploit an endogenous mechanism in dilating the coronary arterial bed. The clinical development of the K_{ATP} channel openers in angina pectoris seems difficult with the notable exception of nicorandil which acts also as a nitrate. The direct effect of the openers on the cardiac myocyte in ischemic conditions is treated in other chapters of the book.

Vascular K_{ATP} channels in a model of insulin-dependent diabetes

Diabetes mellitus is known to predispose the patient for cardiovascular complications such as hypertension, atherosclerosis and thrombosis. When rats are treated with streptozotocin, an insulin-dependent diabetes mellitus (IDDM) develops; in this pathological state the relaxation to the K_{ATP} channel openers cromakalim [67] and aprikalim [68] is impaired in rat aortic strips and cerebral arterioles in vivo. A possible interpretation of these studies is that the expression or the function of vascular K_{ATP} channels may be impaired in this rat model of IDDM. In order to distinguish between these possibilities we have compared the binding of the K_{ATP} channel opener, P1075, as well as its K^+ channel opening and relaxing effects in aortae from streptozotocin (50 mg/kg i.p.)-treated rats and from age-matched controls (Glocker and Quast, unpublished). We found in aortic rings from IDDM rats that:-

(1) the sensitivity and the contractility to noradrenaline were increased,

(2) the acetylcholine-induced (endothelium-dependent) relaxation was slightly enhanced,

(3) the relaxation-concentration curve of the K_{ATP} channel opener P1075 was shifted rightwards and that the maximum attainable relaxation was reduced,

(4) the number of binding sites for ^{3}H-P1075 was increased and the affinity unchanged,

(5) P1075-induced efflux (and thus K^+ channel opening) was augmented at all concentrations tested.

Thus, in IDDM rats the K_{ATP} channel opens normally (if not with increased sensitivity) in response to the opener P1075; however, relaxation to the K_{ATP} channel opener is impaired. This suggests that the relationship between membrane potential and contractility may be changed in this pathological state.

CONCLUSION

Over the last years our knowledge of K^+ channels has progressed tremendously. The two most important points are the cloning of inwardly rectifying K^+ channels and the discovery that native K^+ channels (similar to voltage-dependent Na^+- or Ca^{2+} channels) may contain constituents in addition to the four pore forming α-subunits. Cloning of K_{IR} has revealed a novel superfamily of K^+ channels in addition to the already known voltage-dependent K^+ channels; interestingly the (cardiac) K_{ATP} channel may belong to this new superfamily. The discovery of ß-subunits which govern the inactivation of some K_V channels points at complexities in the structure of native K^+ channels as does the fact that the cloned rcK_{ATP}-1 channel is not sensitive to inhibition by glibenclamide, suggesting that a subunit is missing. Elucidation of the structure of the native K_{ATP} channel will help to elucidate the mechanism by which the K_{ATP} channel openers activate the channel. It is hoped that this progress will accelerate the discovery of novel compounds which modulate this physiologically important channel with improved tissue selectivity.

REFERENCES

1. Hille, B. (1992) Ionic channels of excitable membranes. 2nd edition. Sinauer Associates Inc. Sunderland, Massachusetts.
2. Choquet, D., and Korn, H. (1988) Modulation of voltage-dependent potassium channels in B lymphocytes. *Biochem. Pharmacol.* 7:3797-3802.
3. Jan, L. Y. and Jan, Y. N. (1994) Potassium channels and their evolving gates. *Nature* **371**:119-122.
4. Jan, L. Y., and Jan, Y. N. (1990) A superfamily of ion channels. *Nature* **345**:672.
5. Siegl, P. K. S., Lynch, J. J. (1994) Drugs for prevention of malignant ventricular arrhythmias. *Exp. Opin. Invest. Drugs* **3**:1037-1040.
6. Leonard, R. J., Garcia, M. L. Slaughter, R. S. and Reuben, J. P. (1992) Selective blockers of voltage-gated K^+ channels depolarize human T lymphocytes: mechanism of the antiproliferative effect of charybdotoxin. *Proc. Natl. Acad. Sci. (USA)* **89**:10094-10098.
7. Rettig, J., Heinemann, S. H., Wunder, F., et al. (1994) Inactivation properties of voltage-gated K^+ channels altered by presence of ß-subunit. *Nature* **369**:289-294.
8. Edwards, G., and Weston, A. H., (1994) Effect of potassium channel modulating drugs on isolated smooth muscle. *In: Handbook of Experimental Pharmacology, Vol. 111* (Eds: L. Szekeres and J. G. Papp). Springer, Heidelberg, pp 469-531.
9. McManus, O. B. (1991) Calcium-activated potassium channels: regulation by calcium. *J. Bioenerget. Biomemb.* **23**:537-560.
10. Atkinson, N. S., Robertson, G. A., and Ganetzky, B. (1991) A component of calcium-activated potassium channels encoded by the drosophila slo locus. *Science* **253**:551-555.
11. Adelman, J. P., Shen, K. Z., Kavanaugh, M. P., Warren, R. A., Wu, Y.-N., Lagrutta, A., Bond, C. T., and North, R. A. (1992) Calcium-activated potas-sium channels expressed from cloned complementary DNAs. *Neuron.* **9**:209-216.

12. Butler, A., Tsunoda, S., McCobb, D. P., Wei, A., and Salkoff, L. (1993) mSlo, a complex mouse gene encoding "Maxi" calcium-activated potassium channels. *Science* **261**:221-224.

13. Knaus, H.-G., Folander, K., Garcia-Calvo, M., Garcia, M. L., Kaczorowski.G. J., Smith, M., and Swanson R. (1994) Primary sequence and immunological characterization of ß-subunit of high conductance Ca^{2+}-activated K^{+}channel from smooth muscle. *J. Biol. Chem.* **269**:17274-17278.

14. Olesen, S. P. (1994) Activators of large-conductance Ca^{2+}-dependent K^{+} channels. *Exp. Opin. Invest. Drugs* **3**:1181-1188.

15. Ho, K., Nichols, C. G., Lederer, W. J., Lytton, J., Vassilev, P. M., Kanazirska, M. V., and Hebert S. C. (1993) Cloning and expression of an inwardly rectifying ATP-regulated potassium channel. *Nature* **362**:31-38.

16. Lopatin, A. N., Makhina, E. N., and Nichols C. G. (1994) Potassium channel block by cytoplasmic polyamines as the mechanism of intrinsic rectification. *Nature* **372**:366-369.

17. Kubo, Y., Reuveny, E., Slesinger P. A., Jan, Y. N., and Jan L. Y. (1993) Primary structure and functional expression of a rat G-protein-coupled muscarinic potassium channel. *Nature* **364**:802-806.

18. Ashford, M. L. J., Bond, C.T., Blair, T. A., and Adelman, J. P. (1994) Cloning and functional expression of a rat heart K_{ATP} channel. *Nature* **370**:456-459.

19. Reuveny, E., Slesinger, P. A., and Inglese, J., et al. (1994) Activation of the cloned muscarinic potassium channel by G_i protein ßγ subunits. *Nature* **370**:143-146.

20. Brown, D. A. (1990) G-proteins and potassium currents in neurons. *Annu. Rev. Physiol.* **52**:215-242.

21. Kurachi, Y. (1994) G-Protein control of cardiac potassium channels. *Trends Cardiovasc. Med.* 4:64-69.

22. Ashcroft, S. J. H., and Ashcroft., F. M. (1990) Properties and functions of ATP-sensitive K^{+}-channels. *Cell. Signal.* **2**:197-214.

23. Edwards, G., and Weston, A. H. (1993) The pharmacology of ATP-sensitive K^{+} channels. *Annu. Rev. Pharmacol. Toxicol.* **33**:597-637.

24. Quast, U., Guillon J.-M., and Cavero, I. (1995) Modulation of K^{+} channels:

Pharmacological and therapeutical aspects. *Kluver*, in press

25. Quast, U. (1992) Potassium channel openers: pharmacological and clinical aspects. *Fundam. Clin. Pharmacol.* **107**:945-293.
26. Quast, U., and Cook, N. S. (1989) Moving together: K^+ channel openers and ATP-sensitive K^+ channels. *Trends Pharmacol. Sci.* **10**:431-435.
27. Krapivinsky, G., Gordon, E. A., Wickman, K., Velimirovic, B. Krapivisnky, L. and Clapham, D. E. (1995) The G-protein-gated atrial K^+ channel I_{KACh} is a heteromultimer of two inwardly rectifying K^+-channel proteins. *Nature* **374**:135-141.
28. Schwanstecher, M., Löser, S., Chudziak, F., and Panten, U. (1994) Identification of a 38-kDa high affinity sulfonylurea-binding peptide in insulin-secreting cells and cerebral cortex. *J. Biol. Chem.* **269**:17768-17771.
29. Aguilar-Bryan, L., Clement, J. Nelson, D. A. and Bryon, J. (1995) *Biophys. J.* **69**:A234
30. Escande, D., and Cavero, I. (1992) K^+ channels openers and 'natural' cardioprotection. *Trends Pharmcol. Sci.* **13**:269-272.
31. Cook, N. S., Rudin, M., Pally, C., Blarer, S., and Quast, U. (1993) Effects of the potassium channel openers SDZ-PCO 400 and cromakalim in an in vivo rat model of occlusive arterial disease assessed by ^{31}P-NMR spectroscopy. *J. Vasc. Med. Biol.* **4**: 14-22.
32. Gallin, E. K. (1991) Ion channels in leukocytes. *Physiol. Rev.* **71**:775-811.
33. Haslberger, A., Romanin, C., and Koerber, R. (1992) Membrane potential modulates release of tumor necrosis factor in lipopolysaccharide-stimulated mouse macrophages. *Mol. Biol. Cell* **3**:451-460.
34. Kubo, Y., Baldwin, T. J., Jan, N. Y., and Jan L. Y. (1993) Primary structure and functional expression of a mouse inward rectifier potassium channel. *Nature* **362**:127-133.
35. Davies, P. F., Olesen, S.-P., Clapham, D. E., Morrel, E. M., and Schoen F. J. (1988) Endothelial communication. *Hypertension* **11**:563-572.
36. Newby, A. C., and Henderson, A. H. (1990) Stimulus-secretion coupling in vascular endothelial cells. *Annu. Rev. Physiol.* **52**:661-674.
37. Revest P. A., and Abbot N. J. (1992) Membrane ion channels of endothelial cells. *Trends Pharmacol. Sci.* **13**:404-407.

38. Adams, D. J., Barakeh, F., Laskey, R., and van Breemen, C. (1989) Ion channels and regulation of intracellular calcium in vascular endothelial cells. *FASEB J.***3**:2389-2400.

39. Lückhoff, A., and Busse, R. (1990) Activators of potassium channels enhance calcium influx into endothelial cells as a consequence of potassium currents. *Naunyn-Schmiedeberg's Arch. Pharmacol.* **342**:94-99.

40. Mehrke, G., Pohl, U. and Daut, J. (1991) Effects of vasoactive agonists on the membrane potential of cultured bovine aortic and guinea-pig coronary endothelium. *J. Physiol.* **439**:277-299.

41. Janigro D., West, A. G., Gordon E. L., and Winn, H. R. (1993) ATP-sensitive K^+ channels in rat aorta and brain microvascular endothelial cells. *Cell Physiol.* **34**:C812-C821.

42. Drieu la Rochelle, C., Richard, V., Dubois-Randé, J.-L., Roupie, E., Giudicelli, J. F., Hittinger, L., and Berdeaux, A. (1992) Potassium channel openers dilate large epicardial coronary arteries in conscious dogs by an indirect, endothelium-dependent mechanism. *J. Pharmacol. Exp. Therap.* **263**:1091-1096.

43. Bolton, T. B. and Beech, D. J. (1992) In: *Potassium channel modulators,* Weston, A. H., and Hamilton T. C. (eds). Blackwell Scientific Publications, London, pp 144-180.

44. Edwards, G., and Weston, A. H. (1995) Potassium channels in the regulation of vascular smooth muscle tone. *Kluver*, in press.

45. Nelson, M. T., Patlak, J. B., Worley, J. F., and Standen, N. B. (1990) Calcium channels, potassium channels, and voltage dependence of arterial smooth muscle tone. *Am. J. Physiol.* **259**:C3-C18.

46. Edwards, F. R., and Hirst, G. D. S. (1988) Inward rectification in submucosal arterioles of guinea-pig ileum. *J. Physiol. Lond.* **404**:437-454.

47. Quayle, J. M., McCarron, J. G., Brayden, J. E., and Nelson, M. T. (1993) inward rectifier K^+ currents in smooth muscle cells from rat resistance-sized cerebral arteries. *Am. J. Physiol.* **265**:C1363-C1370.

48. Daut, J., Maier-Rudolph, W., von Beckerath, N., Mehrke, G., Guenther, K., and Goedel-Meinen, L. (1990) Hypoxic dilation of coronary arteries is mediated by ATP-sensitive potassium channels. *Science* **247**:1341-1344.

49. Dart, C., and Standen N. B. (1993) Adenosine-activated potassium current in smooth muscle cells isolated from the pig coronary artery. *J. Physiol (London).* **471**:767-786.

50. Jackson, W. F., König, A., Dambacher, T., and Busse, R. (1993) Prostacyclin-induced vasodilation in rabbit heart is mediated by ATP-sensitive potassium channels. *Am. J. Physiol.* **264**:H238-H243.

51. Quayle, J. M., Bonev, A. D., Brayden, J. E., and Nelson, M. T. (1994) Calcitonin gene-related peptide activated ATP-sensitive K^+ currents in rabbit arterial smooth muscle via proteinkinase. *Am. J. Physiol.* **475** **19**-13.

52. Clapp, L. H., and Gurney, A. M. (1992) ATP-sensitive K^+ channels regulate resting potential of pulmonary arterial smooth muscle cells. *Am. J. Physiol.* **262**:H916-H920.

53. Noack, Th., Edwards, G., Deitmer, P., and Weston, A. H. (1992) Potassium channel modulation by ATP depletion: a comparison with the effects of levcromakalim (BRL 38227). *Br. J. Pharmacol.* **107**:945-955.

54. Silberberg, S. D., and Van Breemen, C. (1992) A potassium current activated by lemakalim and metabolic inhibition in rabbit mesenteric artery. *Pflügers Arch.* **420**: 118-120.

55. Beech, D. J., Zhang, H., Nakao, K., and Bolton, T. B. (1993) K^+ channel activation by nucleoside diphosphates and its inhibition by glibenclamide in vascular smooth muscle cells. *Br. J. Pharmacol.* **110**:573-582.

56. Bray, K. M., and Quast, U. (1992a) A specific binding site for K^+ channel openers in rat aorta. *J. Biol. Chem.* **267**:11689-11692.

57. Quast, U., Bray, K. M., Andres, P. W., Manley, Baumlin, Y., and Dosogne, J. (1993) Binding of the K^+ channel opener [3H]P1075 in rat isolated aorta: relationship to functional effects of openers and blockers. *Mol. Pharmacol.* **43**:474-481.

58. Quast, U. (1993) Do the K^+ channel openers relax smooth muscle by opening K^+ channels? *Trends Pharmacol. Sci.* **14**:332-336.

59. Hamilton, T. C., Weir, S. W., and Weston A. H. (1986) Comparison of the effects of BRL 34915 and verapamil on electrical and mechanical activity in rat portal vein. *Br. J. Pharmacol.* **88**:103-111.

60. Quast, U., and Cook, N. S. (1989) In vitro and in vivo comparison of two

K^+ channel openers, diazoxide and cromakalim, and their inhibition by glibenclamide. *J. Pharmacol. Exp. Ther.* **250**:261-270.

61. Quast, U. (1995) Effects of potassium channel activators in isolated blood vessels. In: *Potassium Channels and their Modulators* (Evans J. et al., eds), Ellis Horwood, in press.

62. Angersbach, D. and Nicholson, C. D. (1988) Enhancement of muscle blood cell flux and pO_2 by cromakalim (BRL 34915) and other compounds enhancing membrane K^+ conductance, but not by Ca^{2+} antagonists or hydralazine, in an animal model of occlusive arterial disease. *Naunyn-Schmiedeberg's Arch. Pharmacol.* **337**:341-346.

63. Randall, M. D., Ujiie, H., and Griffith T. M. (1994) Modulation of vasodilatation to levromakalim by adenosine analogues in the rabbit ear: an explanation for hypoxic augmentation. *Br. J. Pharmacol.* **112**:49-54.

64. Struijker-Boudier, H. A. J., Messing, M. W. J., and van Essen, H. (1992) Preferential small arteriolar vasodilatation by the potassium channel opener, BRL 38227, in conscious spontaneously hypertensive rats. *Eur. J. Pharmacol.* **218**:191-193.

65. Hof, R. P., Quast, U., Cook, N. S. and Blarer, S. (1988) Mechanism of action and systemic and regional hemodynamics of the potassium channel activator BRL34915 and its enantiomers. *Circulation Res.* **62**:679-686.

66. Leenen, F. H. H., Smith, D. L., and Unger, W. P. (1988) Topical minoxidil: cardiac effects in bald man. *Br. J. Clin. Pharmacol.* **26**:481-485.

67. Kamata, K., Miyata, N., and Kasuya, Y. (1989) Functional changes in potassium channels in aortas from rats with streptozotocin-induced diabetes. *Eur. J. Pharmacol.* **166**:319-323.

68. Mayhan, W. G., and Faraci, F. M. (1993) Responses of cerebral arterioles in diabetic rats to activation of ATP-sensitive potassium channels. *Am. J. Physiol.* **265**:H152-H157.

3

ACTIVATION OF ATP-SENSITIVE POTASSIUM CHANNELS: A NOVEL PHARMACOLOGICAL APPROACH TO MYOCARDIAL PROTECTION?

DAVID J HEARSE
Cardiovascular Research, The Rayne Institute, St Thomas' Hospital, London SE1 7EH. UK.

INTRODUCTION:

A number of compounds of widely differing chemical structure have been developed in an attempt to alter the open probability of what has become known as the adenosine triphosphate-sensitive potassium channel (K_{ATP} channel). They include channel openers (such as pinacidil, aprikalim, nicorandil, bimakalim, cromakalim and its active enantiomer levcromakalim) and channel blockers such as glibenclamide, tolbutamide and 5-hydroxydecanoate. They all are able to override the actions of an array of biochemical regulators of channel activity including ATP (an inhibitor of channel opening), adenosine diphosphate, adenosine, fatty acids, lactate, pyruvate and pH (for detailed reviews on the nature of the K_{ATP} channel and its biological and pharmacological control see (1-6)

K_{ATP} channels are found, and have been extensively studied, in many tissues such as smooth muscle, skeletal muscle, brain and pancreas. They are also present in the heart, where they have received considerable attention as a potential new class of therapeutic agent for the control of cardiovascular disease (17-22). It has been argued that K_{ATP} openers or blockers might beneficially modify the consequences of myocardial ischaemia in man, through a variety of possible mechanisms operative at the level of the myocyte and/or the vasculature.

Footnote: This article has been reproduced by permission of the Publishers and the author from Cardiovascular Research *1995; 29: in the press. The advice and discussion of Drs W. Coetzee, M. Shattock, M. Curtis, I. Cavero, G. Gross, G. Grover and L. Clapp are gratefully acknowledged.*

However, the large experimental literature on the cardioprotective properties of these drugs appears conflicting and confusing, with claims that they are variously anti-ischaemic, pro-ischaemic, anti-arrhythmic, pro-arrhythmic or without any effect. In addition, the putative mechanisms by which these drugs exert their various effects are becoming increasingly controversial. This review seeks to identify these areas of controversy and, where possible, to seek a consensus on the properties of this interesting group of pharmacological agents.

ASSESSING THE CARDIOPROTECTIVE EFFECTS OF K_{ATP} MODULATION:

The literature indicates that there are at least nine major variables that need to be taken into account when evaluating the results of different studies. In general, studies can be divided on the basis of: (i) the K_{ATP} channel opener under study and whether or not it was also evaluated in the presence of a K_{ATP} channel blocker, (ii) the species used (most, but not all, studies have been carried out in the dog or the rat), (iii) the route of drug administration (intravenous versus intracoronary), (iv) the dosage and whether it was sufficient to induce a significant shortening of cardiac action potential duration and/or vascular relaxation, (v) whether the drug was given before (as is most common), during or after the induction of ischaemia, (vi) whether the study was in vivo or in vitro, (vii) whether ischaemia was regional or global, (viii) whether reperfusion was instituted and (ix) the chosen end-point for the assessment of injury - a crucial factor in interpreting results and assessing the protective potential of any intervention. In this review, the literature will be divided on the basis of the chosen end-point of injury. In the following section the importance of end-points will be discussed.

End-Points for the Assessment of Injury and Protection:

As will become apparent later, most studies of the K_{ATP} channel and myocardial protection have used either (i) post-ischaemic recovery of contractile function or (ii) infarct size limitation as the end-point. However, in some, diastolic state (contracture) during ischaemia has been used as well as changes in tissue metabolite content, ultrastructure, creatine kinase leakage, susceptibility to ischaemia- and reperfusion-induced arrhythmias and changes in coronary flow and its distribution.

Problems in the Assessment of Injury and Protection:

It is well recognised that the assessment of myocardial injury and its modification is beset by many problems. In the following section a number of these are identified and discussed since they will play an important part in the subsequent evaluation of the literature.

Difficulties in Using Arrhythmias as an End-point: One end-point that is a source of considerable confusion, is the severity of the various arrhythmias that occur during ischaemia or reperfusion. There are three reasons for this: (i) it could be argued that the consequences of K_{ATP} channel activation (shortening of action potential duration) that allegedly help to protect the contractile capacity of the myocyte, might simultaneously increase its susceptibility to arrhythmias, (ii) the failure of some investigators to distinguish between the ability of an intervention to alter the severity (e.g., incidence) as opposed to the time-course (i.e., the time-to-onset) of an arrhythmia and (iii), although not often considered, the possibility that the reduction in the severity of ischaemic injury might paradoxically increase electrical instability. Underlying this last point is the fact that susceptibility to arrhythmias may be greatest in tissue with only a moderate degree of reversible injury. With increasing durations or severities of ischaemia, susceptibility to ischaemia-induced arrhythmias eventually declines since necrotic tissue does not act as a focus of arrhythmogenesis. Thus, interventions that are able to reduce the severity of ischaemic injury (and so delay the onset of necrosis) might occasionally increase the likelihood of arrhythmias originating from within the ischaemic zone. Adding to these problems is the fact that few studies control fully for factors such as heart rate, autonomic tone, collateral flow and the size of the ischaemic zone - all of which can exert a profound effect upon susceptibility to arrhythmias.

Difficulties Arising from the Temporal and Spatial Characteristics of Injury: As reviewed previously (23,24), failure to account for: (i) the temporal and spatial characteristics of evolving infarction, (ii) the major role played by collateral flow (which can vary greatly within hearts, between hearts and between species) and (iii) the highly variable anatomy of the ischaemic zone, has often led to inappropriate, over-optimistic or incorrect assessments of the ability of drugs to reduce infarct size. In this review, only those infarct studies that take these baseline determinants into full account will be considered as providing definitive evidence of the ability of K_{ATP} channel modulating drugs to modify infarct size.

Failing to Distinguish between Modifying the Rate Versus the Extent of Injury or Recovery: Failure to take into account the critical distinction between the undoubted ability of many drugs to slow the *rate* of development of ischaemia-induced injury versus their more questionable ability to achieve a sustained reduction in the *extent* of injury, has confounded the interpretation of many studies in which post-ischaemic recovery of contractile function has been used to assess protection. It is well established (25) that even a short period of myocardial ischaemia, followed by reperfusion, can result in myocardial stunning. In this phenomenon there is no necrosis but, nonetheless, contractile function (and metabolism) may take several hours or days to fully recover. However, so long as sufficient time is allowed, a complete recovery will occur. Whilst the extent of stunning is dependent upon the duration and severity of the preceding ischaemia, it is also thought to be determined by the occurrence of reversible 'reperfusion-induced injury' from which the heart may take considerable time to recover. This review will cite many studies in which K_{ATP} channel openers have been shown to improve the *short term* (15-360 min) recovery of contractile function. It should be stressed, however, that, despite its crucial importance, the design of most of these studies prevents the reader from making a clear distinction between: (i) the ability of the drugs to reduce the extent of necrosis (an event that would lead to a *sustained* improvement in post-ischaemic functional performance - irrespective of the duration of reperfusion) and (ii) their ability to reduce the extent of stunning and so accelerate the *rate* of functional recovery (a transient, but possibly useful, form of protection that would not result in a sustained difference between control and drug-treated hearts). Unfortunately few, if any, studies have incorporated durations of reperfusion that are sufficiently long to allow this crucial distinction to be made. Ideally, protocols should allow reperfusion for 2-4 days before function is assessed and infarct size is measured. Unfortunately, this is only possible in in-vivo models.

REVIEW OF K_{ATP} CHANNEL OPENERS AND POST-ISCHAEMIC CONTRACTILE FUNCTION:

With few exceptions, studies employing contractile function during reperfusion as an end-point for the assessment of injury and protection fall into two distinct categories: (i) those carried out in vivo, most of which employ the open-chest anaesthetised dog with brief (usually 15 min) *regional* ischaemia, using the recovery of segmental wall function as the end-point of protection and (ii) those carried out in vitro, most of which involve the use of the crystalloid perfused rat heart and severe (25-30 min of zero flow) *global* ischaemia, using either pump function (cardiac output in working preparations) or pressure development (in Langerdorff models) as the end-point. In both instances, it is tempting to equate the end-point with myocardial 'stunning' (particularly in dog studies in which classical stunning protocols are employed). However, this term should be applied with caution since stunning is a fully reversible phenomenon (no necrosis) from which the heart may take several hours or days to recover. As mentioned above, unless recoveries are measured over these extended times, it is impossible to determine definitively whether the improved (but nonetheless incomplete) recovery of segmental wall function seen in most studies after 3 or 4 h of reperfusion is due to an acceleration in the recovery from stunning, a reduction of necrosis or both.

Efficacy: Can K_{ATP} Channel Openers Improve Post-ischaemic Functional Recovery?

Figure 1 shows the results of a dog study by Grover et al (26) in which cromakalim (for this and doses for all other studies see Table 1) was given by intracoronary infusion for 15 min before the onset and throughout 15 min of regional ischaemia and 180 min of reperfusion. Segment shortening decreased to negative values during ischaemia in both control and drug-treated hearts. During reperfusion, control hearts exhibited very poor recovery of function such that, by the end of the reperfusion period, segment shortening was less than 5% of its pre-ischaemic control value. By contrast, in hearts treated with cromakalim, striking protection was observed such that segment shortening at the end of the reperfusion was greater than 45% of its pre-ischaemic control value. In a similar dog study from the same laboratory, D'Alonzo et al (27) gave a higher (x10) intracoronary dose of cromakalim, again administered 15 min before and throughout 15 min of regional ischaemia and 180 min of reperfusion; this improved post-ischaemic segment shortening from less than 15% to more than 80% of its pre-ischaemic control.

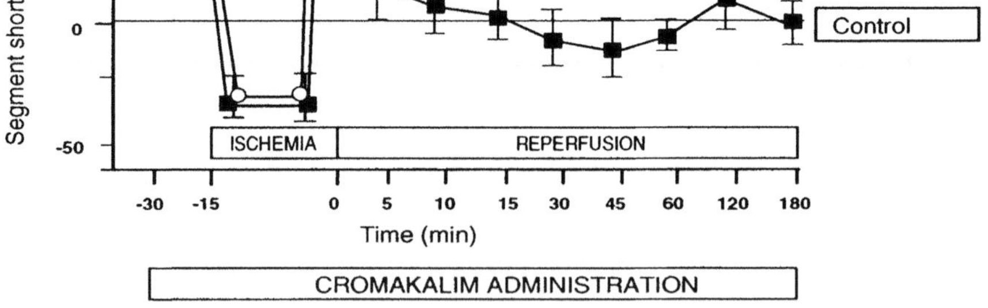

Figure 1: Illustration of the ability of a K_{ATP} channel opener (cromakalim), when administered before regional ischaemia (15 min) and reperfusion (180 min), to enhance post-ischaemic recovery of contractile function in the dog heart. This figure is based on the work of Grover et al [26].

Table 1. K_{ATP} channel openers and post-ischaemic function: species, drugs, doses and duration of ischaemia and reperfusion used by various investigators (i.c. = intracoronary, i.v. = intravenous).

AUTHOR	REFERENCE	SPECIES	DRUG	DOSE	ISCHAEMIA	REPERFUSION
Auchampach et al	[32]	dog	nicorandil	100µg/kg + 25µg/kg/min (i.v.)	15 min	180 min
Auchampach et al	[33]	dog	aprikalim	10µg/kg + 0.1µg/kg/min (i.v.)	15 min	180 min
Cohen et al	[48]	rabbit	aprikalim	100µmol/l	20 min	-
Cole et al	[35]	guinea pig	pinacidil	1 - 10µmol/l	20 - 30 min	60 min
D'Alonzo et al	[27]	dog	cromakalim	1.0µg/kg/min (i.c.)	15 min	180 min
Galiñanes et al	[45]	rat	levcromakalim	10µmol/l	20 - 35 min	40 min
Gross et al	[28]	dog	nicorandil	100µg/kg + 25µg/kg/min (i.v.)	30 min	180 min
Gross et al	[29]	dog	nicorandil	25µg/kg/min (i.v.)	15 min	180 min
Gross et al	[30]	dog	nicorandil	25µg/kg/min (i.v.)	15 min	180 min
Gross et al	[31]	rat	nicorandil	7µmol/l	20 min	30 min
Gross et al	[31]	dog	bimakalim	3µg/kg (i.v.)	15 min	180 min
Gross et al	[31]	dog	nicorandil	100µg/kg + 25µg/kg/min (i.v.)	15 min	180 min
Gross et al	[31]	dog	nicorandil	25µg/kg/min or 100µg/kg + 25µg/kg/min	15 min	180 min
Grover et al	[26]	dog	cromakalim	0.1µg/kg/min (i.c.)	15 min	180 min
Grover et al	[26]	dog	nicorandil	0.3µg/kg/min (i.c.)	15 min	180 min
Grover et al	[36]	rat	cromakalim	1 - 100µmol/l	25 min	30 min
Grover et al	[39]	rat	aprikalim	1 - 100µmol/l	25 min	30 min
Grover et al	[40]	rat	cromakalim	7µmol/l	25 min	30 min
Grover et al	[41]	rat	(+) and (-) cromakalim	0.3 - 100µmol/l	25 min	30 min
Grover et al	[42]	rat	pinacidil	1 - 100µmol/l	25 min	30 min
Grover et al	[42]	rat	cromakalim	1 - 7µmol/l	25 min	30 min
Grover et al	[26]	dog	nicorandil	30µg/kg/min (i.v.)	15 min	180 min
Grover et al	[49]	rat	cromakalim	1 - 100µmol/l	25 min	30 min
Grover et al	[26]	dog	cromakalim	0.1µg/kg/min (i.c.)	15 min	180 min
Grover et al	[26]	rat	nicorandil	10 - 300µmol/l	25 min	30 min
Haneda et al	[52]	rat	nicorandil	50 - 150µmol/l	20 min	20 min
Irie et al	[46]	dog	nicorandil	2 - 10mg/l	120 min	120 min
McCullough et al	[37]	rat	cromakalim	0.05 - 1.0µmol/l	25 min	30 min
Mitani et al	[51]	rat	nicorandil	100 - 200µmol/l	30 min	30 min
Ohta et al	[50]	rat	nicorandil	10 - 100µmol/l	25 min	30 min
Pieper et al	[53]	rat	nicorandil	0.7 - 7µmol/l	30 min	30 min
Qiu et al	[54]	rat	nicorandil	2 -100µmol/l	20 - 30 min	30 min
Sargent et al	[38]	rat	cromakalim	7µmol/l	25 min	30 min
Sugimoto et al	[47]	guinea pig	nicorandil	1000µmol/l	120 min (hypoxia)	60 min
Udvary et al	[34]	rabbit	cromakalim	10 - 300µg/kg (i.v.)	5 min (pacing)	-

Can Protection be Obtained with all K_{ATP} Channel Openers?

Numerous studies have shown that improvements in post-ischaemic recovery can be obtained with all agents in this class. Furthermore, the extent of the protection appears to be remarkably similar, despite the use of structurally dissimilar agents (some of which, such as nicorandil with its nitrate moiety, have important secondary properties), given at different concentrations, sometimes by different routes. Thus, for example, Gross et al (21,28-31) using either anaesthetised or conscious dogs with 10 min (31), 15 min (28-31) or 30 min (30) of regional ischaemia and 3 - 6 h of reperfusion, reported that intravenous nicorandil, administered 10 min (30), 15 min (28,31) or 30 min (29,31) prior to and throughout the ischaemic period (and being either not present during the reperfusion period or present only for the first 30 min of reperfusion), improved the post ischaemic recovery of segment shortening in every instance. Despite the multitude of protocol variations, the protection was similar in all cases, with segmental shortening at the end of reperfusion being improved from less than 20% to greater than 75% of its pre-ischaemic control value. Gross et al (31) also studied the effects of bimakalim given as a bolus to anaesthetised dogs 15 min before occlusion and observed good protection of post-ischaemic function. Auchampach et al (32), using a near identical protocol to that of Gross et al (31), reported that nicorandil conferred a similar improvement of post-ischaemic segment shortening. Auchampach et al (33), using the dog, again with a similar protocol, reported that intravenous aprikalim improved recovery from less than 10% to greater than 80%. Grover et al (26), in addition to studying cromakalim (see previous section), also investigated intravenous nicorandil, administered 15 min prior to and throughout 15 min of ischaemia and 180 min of reperfusion and found that it improved the post-ischaemic recovery of segment shortening from less than 5% to greater than 40%. It is important to note that, in all of the studies cited thus far, the drugs were administered *well before* the onset of ischaemia. It is also important to recognise that the duration of drug treatment varied greatly between studies such that in some instances treatment was carried on throughout the experiment (i.e., until the end of reperfusion), whereas in others the treatment was discontinued part way through the reperfusion period whilst, in others, the treatment was confined to the ischaemic period or the period leading up to the induction of ischaemia.

Do K_{ATP} Channel Openers Afford Protection in all Species?

Although most studies with regional ischaemia have been carried out using canine hearts, there have been a considerable number of studies in other species confirming that the dog is not unique in benefiting from the protective effects of K_{ATP} channel openers. Thus, Udvary et al (34) used the rabbit heart with pacing-induced ischaemia to demonstrate that intravenous cromakalim was able to attenuate increases in diastolic pressure from greater than 25 to less than 10 mmHg. Cole et al (35) subjected isolated guinea pig right ventricular wall preparations to 20-30 min of global ischaemia and 60 min of reperfusion and demonstrated that pinacidil, given for 15 min before ischaemia but not during reperfusion, improved the recovery of post-ischaemic function from less than 40% to greater than 85%. In several studies, Grover and colleagues (36-41) have used the isolated perfused rat heart with 25 min of global ischaemia and 30 min of reperfusion to demonstrate that pinacidil, cromakalim or RP-52891 (aprikalim), added to the perfusate for 10 min immediately prior to ischaemia (but not during reperfusion), improved the post-ischaemic recovery of left ventricular developed pressure from less than 25 mmHg to greater than 80mmHg with pinacidil; from less than 30% to greater than 95% with cromakalim and from less than 30% to greater than 70% with aprikalim. In one of these studies, Grover et al (41) compared the two enantiomers of cromakalim in the rat heart and demonstrated stereospecificity with much higher protective potency with the (-)-enantiomer (levcromakalim) which is the enantiomer with the highest potency as a K_{ATP} channel opener.

Specificity: Is the K_{ATP} Channel Necessarily Involved?

A question that obviously arises is whether all members of this diverse group of drugs (particularly nicorandil with its additional nitrate property) necessarily achieve their protective effects by means of a mechanism that involves the K_{ATP} channel. This has been well investigated in a number of the experimental preparations described above. In each instance, the ability of a K_{ATP} channel blocker to abolish or attenuate the protection afforded by the K_{ATP} channel opener has been assessed. Thus, Auchampach et al

(32,33), in dog heart studies with 15 min of regional ischaemia and 180 min of reperfusion, have shown (Figure 2) that nicorandil and aprikalim, administered intravenously 15 min prior to and throughout the period of ischemia (but not during the reperfusion period), improved post-ischaemic segment shortening from its drug-free control value of less than 20% to greater than 75%. However, whilst glibenclamide alone (0.3 mg/kg, given as a bolus 30 min before the onset of ischaemia) was shown to have no significant effect on post-ischaemic contractile dysfunction, it totally abolished the protection afforded by the K_{ATP} channel opener.

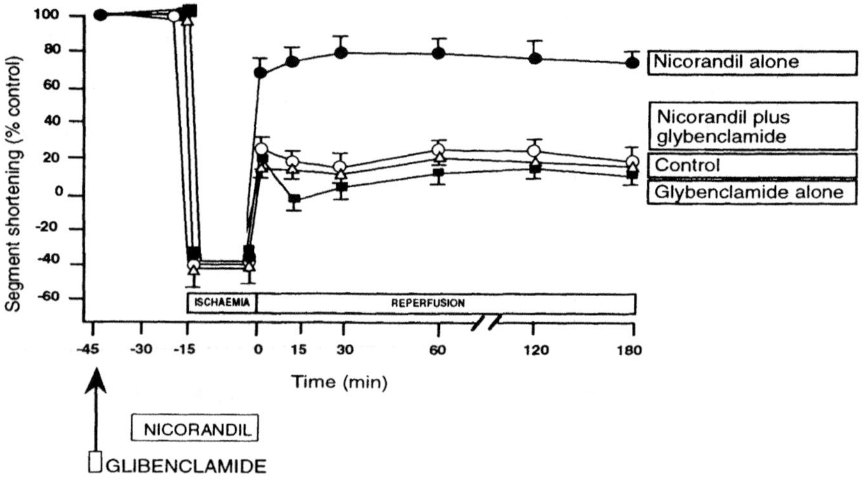

Figure 2: Illustration of the ability of a K_{ATP} channel blocker (glibenclamide, given prior to ischaemia) to attenuate the ability of a K_{ATP} channel opener (nicorandil) to improve the post-ischaemic recovery of function in the dog heart subjected to 15 min of regional ischaemia and 180 min of reperfusion. Given alone, glibenclamide had no significant effect on functional recovery. This figure is based on the work of Auchampach et al [32]

Similar findings have been reported for cromakalim in the rabbit (34) and for pinacidil in the guinea pig heart (35). In the latter study, glibenclamide alone was shown to be detrimental to post-ischaemic functional recovery, however, it was used at a high concentration (10 µmol/l). Grover and colleagues (36-40,42,43) have also reported a series of studies in rat hearts in which the K_{ATP} channel blockers glibenclamide (1 µmol/l or 1 mg/kg) or 5-hydroxydecoanoate (100-300 mmol/l) were shown to reverse the protection afforded by cromakalim, aprikalim, pinacidil and BMS-180448. In a dog-heart study, Auchampach et al (33) used glibenclamide (1 mg/kg) and tolbutamide (100 mg/kg) and demonstrated that the administration of the blockers alone, 30 min prior to ischaemia, resulted in a significant worsening of post-ischaemic function. Finally, Sargent et al (38) undertook an important study aimed at assessing the specificity of glibenclamide. Using isolated rat hearts with 25 min of ischaemia and 30 min of reperfusion, with post-ischaemic functional recovery and enzyme leakage as indices of protection, they showed that although calcium antagonists, sodium channel blockers and calmodulin antagonists had similar cardioprotective properties to cromakalim, glibenclamide could only attenuate the protection afforded by the K_{ATP} channel opener. They also demonstrated that the protection afforded by cromakalim could not be prevented by blockers of other potassium channels. Unless the ability of glibenclamide to block the K_{ATP} channel is in some way lost during ischaemia (44) then, taken together, the findings described in this section provide strong evidence that K_{ATP} channel openers protect the myocardium by means of a mechanism that specifically involves the K_{ATP} channel.

K_{ATP} Channel Openers and Hyperkalaemic Cardioplegia:

A number of studies have, in addition to assessing the ability of glibenclamide to block K_{ATP} channel-mediated protection, determined whether exogenously increasing extracellular potassium levels influences the protection afforded by K_{ATP} channel openers. They have employed hyperkalaemic cardioplegic solutions to elevate extracellular potassium levels, with the primary objective of determining whether K_{ATP}

channel openers offered any prospect for enhancing the protective properties of these solutions. These studies have shed some light (and also some controversy) on the suggestion that K_{ATP} channel-mediated protection may be related to the cardioplegic properties of these drugs. Thus, Galiñanes et al (45), using isolated rat hearts with 20 min of global ischaemia and 40 min of reperfusion, demonstrated that lemakalim (levcromakalim) treatment (given 2 min before ischaemia) resulted in a marked improvement in the post-ischaemic recovery of left ventricular developed pressure (from 49±7 to 65±3%). In the same study, hearts receiving glibenclamide alone recovered in an identical manner (46±4%) to untreated hearts (again, questioning whether, at the concentration studied (10 μmol/l), glibenclamide is pro-ischaemic). However, when the studies were repeated with high potassium (16 mmol/l) cardioplegia incorporated into the protocol (2 min infusion immediately prior to ischaemia), the addition of either lemakalim or glibenclamide, to the cardioplegic solution, was without effect in terms of post-ischaemic functional recovery. It appeared that the protective effects of the K_{ATP} channel opener were rendered redundant by the simultaneous use of potassium cardioplegia. This lack of an additive effect led Galiñanes et al (45) to speculate that the mechanism of protection of lemakalim might be related to its ability to shorten the action potential and thus exert a cardioplegic protective effect by hastening mechanical arrest and conserving limited energy supplies for subsequent recovery. However, this possibility was somewhat confounded by the author's observations that, although lemakalim reduced slightly the mean time-to-mechanical arrest (128±5 vs 103±2 s), it *increased* time-to-electrical arrest from its control value of 241±30 to 509±161 s). Irie (46) also reported the absence of an additive effect when a K_{ATP} channel opener was added to cardioplegia, this time in a dog-heart study. Nicorandil was added to a cold (4°C) cardioplegic solution that was infused (10-20 ml/kg) into dog hearts in vivo just before, and once every 30 min throughout, a 120 min period of hypothermic (14-17°C) global ischaemia and 120 min of reperfusion. No significant protection was observed as measured by the recovery of left ventricular developed pressure, cardiac output or heart rate. In considering this study, it is important to recognise the possibility that the coincident use of hypothermia may have reduced the ability of the drug to promote K_{ATP} channel opening.

The conclusions of Galiñanes et al (45) and Irie (46) are contradicted in part by the study of Sugimoto et al (47) who used a hypoxic and reoxygenated guinea pig-muscle preparation to determine whether nicorandil pretreatment and/or combination with cardioplegia could afford protection as assessed by the recovery of developed tension after 120 min of hypothermic (20∞C) hypoxia. In both instances, a substantial protective effect was demonstrated and furthermore this could be attenuated by concurrent administration of glibenclamide (1μmol/l). Cohen et al (48) also studied K_{ATP} channel openers in the context of cardioplegia and global ischaemia. Using the isolated rabbit heart, they compared the post-ischaemic recovery of developed pressure in hearts that were subjected to 20 min of zero flow ischaemia with or without pre-ischaemic perfusion for 1-2 min with a high concentration of aprikalim. This drug improved the recovery after 30 min of reperfusion from 58±4 to 101±8% of its pre-ischaemic control value. Clearly, additional studies are required before the role of K_{ATP} channel openers in cardioplegia can be fully established.

Dose-response Characteristics of Protection:

Although cost and logistics often preclude detailed dose-response studies in large animals such as the dog, small mammalian preparations, either in vivo or in vitro, readily allow such characterisation. Figure 3 shows the results of a study taken from the work of Grover et al (36,41,49) where the (+)- and (-)-enantiomers of cromakalim were added to the perfusate of isolated rat hearts 10 min before a 25 min period of global ischaemia and 30 min of reperfusion. A clear dose-dependency was demonstrated with the recovery of post-ischaemic left ventricular developed pressure progressively increasing from less than 25 to greater than 75 mmHg. Grover et al (39,42,43) have also reported dose-response studies with other K_{ATP} channel openers including aprikalim, pinacidil and BMS-180448. Dose-response studies in rabbits have been reported by Udvary et al (34) for cromakalim and by Cohen et al (48) for aprikalim.

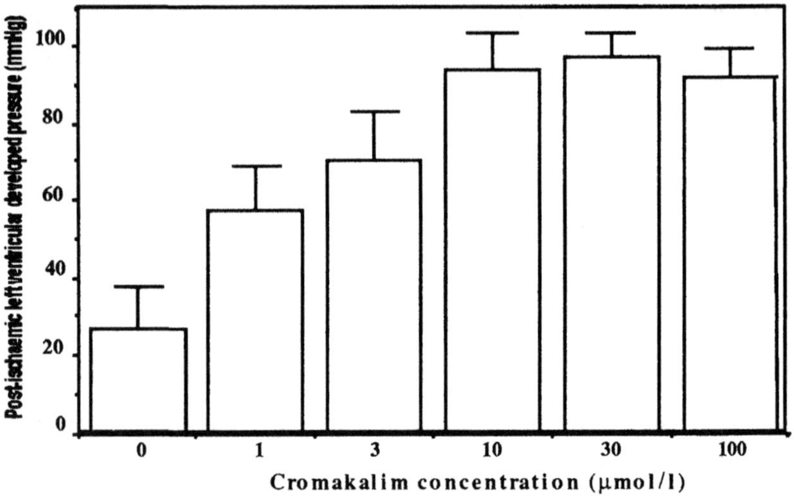

Figure 3: *Dose-response characteristics for the ability of a K_{ATP} channel opener (cromakalim, given before the onset of ischaemia) to improve the post-ischaemic recovery of contractile function in rat hearts that had been subjected to 25 min of global ischaemia and 30 min of reperfusion. This figure is based on the work of Grover et al (36)*

Route of Administration:

As is apparent from the above results, protection can usually be demonstrated when the drug is given either by the intravenous or the intracoronary route. However, in a frequently cited but controversial paper, Grover et al (26) reported a dog study in which nicorandil was given 15 min before and throughout 15 min of regional ischaemia and 180 min of reperfusion. When the drug was given by the intravenous route, good protection was observed with post-ischaemic segment shortening improving from its drug-free control value of less than 5% to greater than 40%. However, when given by the intracoronary route, no significant protection was observed. The authors suggested that this might indicate that, in their study at least, protection was dependent largely on the systemic effects of the drug and was independent of the K_{ATP} channel. However, the attribution of protection to peripheral effects seems unlikely since K_{ATP} channel openers have been effective in isolated heart preparations in which peripheral factors cannot be involved. It is also noteworthy that in the same study, with an identical protocol to that used for nicorandil, Grover et al (26) were able to demonstrate efficacy with intracoronary administration of cromakalim. In commenting on this study, Richer et al (8) pointed out that the infused intracoronary dose of nicorandil was only one hundredth of that chosen for the intravenous dose and only three times larger than the cromakalim dose. They argued that, since nicorandil was ten times less potent than cromakalim, any study designed to compare the two drugs and the two routes of administration should have employed larger doses of nicorandil.

Timing of Administration: When are the Drugs Active?

In all studies cited thus far, the K_{ATP} channel openers or blockers were administered *well before* the onset of ischaemia. Clearly, in clinical practice, the feasibility of administering an anti-ischaemic agent *before* the onset of an ischaemic episode may not always be possible. This consideration was undoubtedly the driving force for a series of studies that have assessed the ability of these drugs to protect the heart when administered *after* the onset of ischaemia. These studies were certainly also influenced by the desire to understand whether the mechanism of protection was primarily operative before or during the episode of ischaemia or even during reperfusion. The latter possibility reflected an interest in whether these drugs were able to attenuate 'reperfusion-induced injury'. In an important study, Auchampach et al (33), administered aprikalim intravenously to dogs subjected to 15 min regional ischaemia and 180 min of reperfusion. The drug was given either 15 min before ischaemia or immediately before reperfusion. As the results displayed in Figure 4 clearly show, late administration of aprikalim was without any significant effect, suggesting that its protective mechanism was operative either before or during the ischaemic episode. As is discussed below, studies in which infarct size was used as an end-point, have allowed further dissection of the time-course of drug action. The findings of Auchampach et al (33) in the dog heart provide valuable support to the study by Grover et al (40) in which cromakalim was given to isolated perfused rat hearts either 10 min before the onset of 25 min ischaemia and 30 min reperfusion or 2 min before the onset of reperfusion. Whilst pre-ischaemic administration improved the post-ischaemic recovery of left ventricular developed pressure from 17±2 mmHg to 81±5 mmHg, administration just prior to reperfusion was without significant effect (36±15 mmHg).

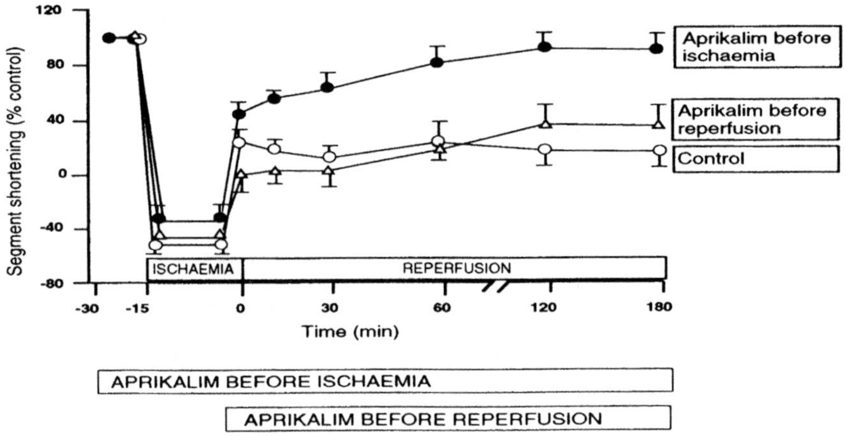

Figure 4: *Illustration of the importance of the time of administration of a K_{ATP} channel blocker in relation to the protection of post-ischaemic recovery of function. When administered to dog hearts before 15 min of regional ischaemia and 180 min of reperfusion, aprikalim afforded striking protection, however, when administered just before reperfusion no protection was observed. This figure is based on the work of Auchampach et al* [33].

Are All Studies of the Effects of K_{ATP} Channel Openers Positive?

Any review of the literature would be imbalanced if it failed to discuss negative studies. In this connection, it is clear that investigations of the protective properties of K_{ATP} channel openers are by no means universally positive. However, it is of interest to note that most of the negative studies appear to be confined to those with protocols that employed the rat heart with global ischaemia and nicorandil as the drug of choice. Thus, Ohta et al (50), Mitani et al (51), Haneda et al (52) and Pieper et al (53) all used isolated rat hearts perfused with nicorandil at concentrations ranging from 1 to 1000 µmol/l.

They all administered the drug before 20-30 min periods of low-flow or zero-flow ischaemia and, unless exceptionally high doses were used (50), failed to observe sustained or substantial improvement in the post-ischaemic recovery of function when measured after 20-30 min of reperfusion (although Pieper et al did observe protection early in the reperfusion period). These findings are open to a number of explanations including: (i) the atypical electrophysiological characteristics of the rat heart (with its very short action potential), (ii) the doses employed (although some were high compared with studies in other species, Grover et al (26) have reported that while nicorandil failed to afford significant protection in the isolated rat heart with doses of up to 100 μmol/l, a dose of 300 μmol/l did result in the recovery of left ventricular developed pressure improving from less than 25% to almost 80%), (iii) the fact that in the low-flow studies at least, any potassium that accumulated during ischaemia (that might contribute to the protective mechanism) may be washed out and (iv) in the case of nicorandil, the ability to reduce peripheral vascular resistance (not operative in an isolated-heart preparation) may be crucial to its profound cardioprotective properties in the in-vivo preparations described above. In connection with this last point Grover et al (26) noted that nicorandil failed to protect the heart when administered by the intracoronary route - a finding the authors attributed to the importance of systemic factors in the mechanism of action of the drug. The nitrate property that distinguishes nicorandil from other drugs in this class, might be an important consideration in assessing these findings. However, not all isolated rat heart studies with nicorandil have been negative, Qiu et al (54) reported a small degree of protection when the drug was given as a *continuous* low-flow infusion during ischaemia.

Complications: Do K_{ATP} Channel Openers Increase Susceptibility to Arrhythmias?

As will be discussed below, theoretical arguments can be advanced to support the possibility that K_{ATP} channel opening drugs might be pro-arrhythmic during ischaemia as a consequence of their ability to shorten action potential duration (especially when used at high concentrations). Whilst it is not the objective of this review to discuss the arrhythmogenesis issue in detail, it should be noted that a number of studies, in which post-ischaemic functional recovery was the primary end-point, have also contained results pertaining to arrhythmias. Thus, in a dose-response study with cromakalim, given to the isolated rat heart only for 10 min before 25 min of global ischaemia and 30 min of reperfusion, Grover et al (36) reported excellent protection in terms of post-ischaemic functional recovery but, at the optimal concentration (7 μmol/l), the drug increased the number of hearts fibrillating during reperfusion from 29% (5/17) in the control group to 59% (10/17). In this study, glibenclamide (1 μmol/l) prevented the pro-fibrillatory effects of cromakalim (0/5). Interestingly, in the same paper, Grover et al (36) reported a positive effect of cromakalim on infarct size in the dog heart and observed that the drug exerted an *anti*-arrhythmic effect (see below). These apparently conflicting results might, as will be discussed later, be explained on the basis of: (i) the use of global ischaemia in the rat and regional ischaemia in the dog, (ii) species differences in action potential duration which is very short in the rat compared to other species and (iii) whether the arrhythmias were re-entrant or triggered. In another study in the rat, Qiu et al (54) gave nicorandil to isolated hearts 3 min before 20 min of ischaemia and 10 min of reperfusion and observed a 50% incidence of ventricular fibrillation in the drug-treated hearts and 0% in the controls. There was also a drug-induced increase in the severity of ventricular tachycardia and other non-sinus rhythms. Cohen et al (48), using the isolated, globally ischaemic (20 min) rabbit heart, were able to show that a brief exposure to aprikalim greatly improved the post-ischaemic recovery of contractile function. However, they also reported that it increased the incidence of reperfusion-induced ventricular fibrillation from 20% to 60%. In a recent prospective randomised study using the isolated rat heart, Rees and Curtis (55) found that neither RP-49356 (10 μmol/l) nor gliblenclamide (10 μmol/l) affected the incidence of ventricular fibrillation during regional ischaemia, despite exerting characteristic effects on coronary flow (increased by RP-49356) and QT interval (widened from 154$\pm$12 ms to 203$\pm$20 ms by glibenclamide and shortened by RP-49356 to 123$\pm$6 ms). However, when used in combination, the drugs caused an unexpected reduction in the incidence of ventricular fibrillation (from 100% to 25%). These investigators attributed this action to a K_{ATP} channel-independent effect of glibenclamide that had been unmasked by the presence of RP-49356. As stressed above, there have been very few prospective studies of this type in which arrhythmias have been selected as the primary end-point; clearly, more studies (particularly in large animals) are needed.

SUMMARY OF THE EFFECTS OF K_{ATP} CHANNEL OPENERS ON THE RECOVERY OF POST-ISCHAEMIC CONTRACTILE FUNCTION:

There is strong evidence that all K_{ATP} channel openers (including nicorandil) can reduce 'stunning' in dog hearts with *regional* ischaemia, provided the drugs are administered *before* the onset of ischaemia. The drugs appear to be without effect if given at the time of reperfusion. The protection can be attenuated by the K_{ATP} channel blocker glibenclamide, thus suggesting the specific involvement of the ATP-sensitive potassium channel. With some exceptions (33,35), glibenclamide alone does not appear to exacerbate post-ischaemic contractile dysfunction, an observation that questions whether, in unmodified ischaemia, K_{ATP} channels are necessarily always open. In rats, rabbits and guinea pigs with *global* ischaemia, most K_{ATP} channel openers, provided that they are given before ischaemia, improve, in a dose-dependent manner, the post-ischaemic recovery of function. This protection can also be abolished by glibenclamide. Most, but not all, isolated *rat*-heart studies with nicorandil show little protection unless very high concentrations of the drug are used. Finally, in the rat heart, some K_{ATP} channel openers appear to exert a pro-arrhythmic effect, which appears to be preventable by the administration of a K_{ATP} channel blocker.

REVIEW OF K_{ATP} CHANNEL OPENERS AND MYOCARDIAL INFARCT SIZE LIMITATION:

The great majority of studies on the ability of K_{ATP} channel openers to influence the evolution of myocardial infarction have been in the dog heart, usually with 60-120 min of regional ischaemia and up to 5 h of reperfusion. In assessing these and other studies, it is crucial to appreciate that the methodology for infarct sizing can be fraught with artefacts and the findings can easily be misinterpreted (23,24). Any study that fails to measure and take account of critical baseline determinants of infarct size (such as collateral flow and risk zone size) or which employs insufficient numbers of animals must be interpreted with considerable caution. In addition, any study with unrealistic expectations (such as those involving very long periods of ischaemia or those in which reperfusion is not initiated) should also be treated with similar reservations.

Efficacy: Can K_{ATP} Channel Openers Limit the Size of an Evolving Infarct?

A number of well designed investigations have provided convincing evidence that virtually every K_{ATP} channel opener studied is able to slow the progression of ischaemic injury and the development of necrosis such that, at the time of reperfusion, more tissue is available for salvage. Figure 5 shows the results from studies of Grover et al (36,40,49) in which cromakalim (for this and doses for all other studies see Table 2) was infused by the intracoronary route into dog hearts starting 10 min before and continuing throughout both 90 min of regional ischaemia and 5 h of reperfusion. Infarct size, measured as a percentage of the ischaemic risk zone, was more than halved from 60±7% to 25±5%. Grover et al [36] also reported that the frequency of ectopic beats and the proportion of animals with ventricular fibrillation was significantly *reduced* in the cromakalim group

Table 2. K_{ATP} openers and infarct size: species, drugs, doses and durations of ischaemia and reperfusion used by various investigators (i.c. = intracoronary, i.v. = intravenous).

AUTHOR	REFERENCE	SPECIES	DRUG	DOSE	ISCHAEMIA	REPERFUSION
Auchampach et al	[59]	dog	aprikalim	10µg/kg + 0.1µg/kg/min (i.v.)	90 min	5 h
Auchampach et al	[60]	dog	bimakalim	3µg/kg + 0.1µg/kg/min (i.v.)	90 min	5 h
Endo et al	[64]	dog	nicorandil	100µg/kg + 30µg/kg/min	360 min	0
Gross et al	[56]	dog	aprikalim	10µg/kg + 0.1µg/kg/min (i.v.)	60 min	5 h
Gross et al	[30]	dog	nicorandil	100µg/kg + 25µg/kg/min (i.v.)	120 min	30 min
Gross et al	[31]	dog	nicorandil	100µg/kg + 25µg/kg/min (i.v.)	120 min	30 min
Gross et al	[31]	dog	bimakalim	3µg/kg + 0.1µg/kg/min (i.v.)	120 min	30 min
Grover et al	[36]	dog	cromakalim	0.1µg/kg/min (i.c.)	90 min	5 h
Grover et al	[49]	dog	cromakalim	0.1µg/kg/min (i.c.)	90 min	5 h
Grover et al	[40]	dog	cromakalim	0.1µg/kg/min (i.c.)	90 min	5 h
Grover et al	[40]	dog	pinadicil	0.9µg/kg/min (i.c.)	90 min	5 h
Grover et al	[43]	dog	BMS-180448	50µg/kg/min (i.v.)	90 min	5 h
Imai et al	[68]	dog	pinacidil	4.0±0.6µg/kg/min (i.v.)	240 min	20 h
Kitzen et al	[66]	dog	cromakalim	0.2µg/kg/min (i.c or i.v.)	90 min	5 h
Kitzen et al	[66]	dog	celikalim	0.2µg/kg/min (i.c. or i.v.)	90 min	5 h
Yao et al	[63]	dog	bimakalim	0.1-10µg/kg (i.c.)	60 min	4 h
Lamping et al	[57]	dog	nicorandil	100µg/kg + 25µg/kg/min (i.v.)	120 min	30 min
Mizumura et al	[58]	dog	nicorandil	100µg/kg + 10µg/kg/min (i.v.)	60 min	3 h
Mizumura et al	[65]	dog	bimakalim	1µg/kg + 0.05µg/kg/min (i.v.)	60 min	3 h
Rohman et al	[61]	pig	bimakalim	3µg/kg + 0.1µg/kg/min (i.v.)	60 min	120 min
Sakamoto et al	[67]	dog	pinacidil	4µg/kg/min (i.v.)	240 min	20 h
Smallwood et al	[69]	dog	pinacidil	1µg/kg/min (i.c.)	90 min	5 h
Smallwood et al	[69]	dog	3 pyridyl-pinacidil	0.25-1.0µg/kg/min (i.c.)	90 min	5 h
Toombs et al	[62]	rabbit	cromakalim	20µg/kg (i.v.)	30 min	2 h

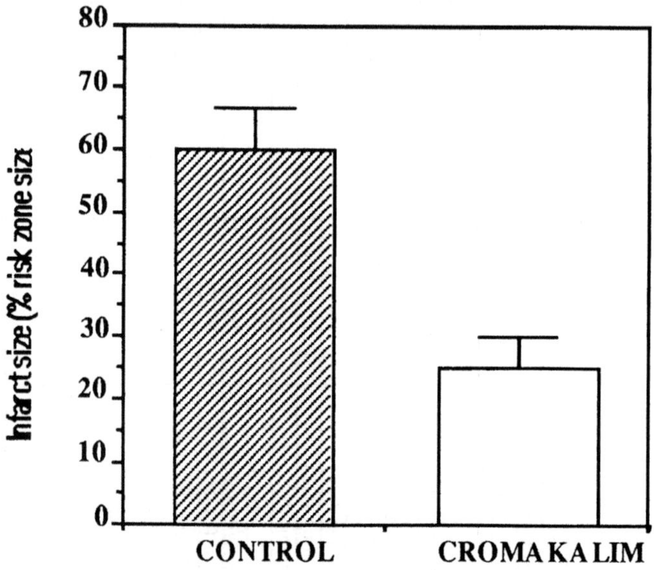

Figure 5: *Illustration of the ability of a K_{ATP} channel opener (cromakalim), when administered prior to regional ischaemia (50 min) and reperfusion (5 h) to limit the size of an evolving infarct in the dog heart. This figure is based on the work of Grover et al (49).*

(1/9 versus 6/11). Recently, Grover et al (43) have also reported that BMS-180448 (a K_{ATP} channel opener devoid of vasodilator activity), given intravenously to dogs 10 min before and for the first 30 min of a 90 min period of ischaemia, reduced infarct size, measured at the end of 5 h of reperfusion, from its control value of greater than 50% to approximately 25%. Similar halvings of infarct size in dogs with other K_{ATP} channel openers have been reported by Gross et al (56) who demonstrated that aprikalim, given intravenously, 10 min before and continuing throughout both 60 min of regional ischaemia and 5 h of reperfusion, reduced infarct size from 28±6% to 13±3%. Gross et al (30,57) also reported that intravenous nicorandil reduced infarct size, in dog hearts subjected to 120 min of regional ischaemia and 30 min of reperfusion, from 38±5% to 19±3%. The same group(58) also gave nicorandil intravenously 15 min before and throughout a shorter period (60 min) of regional ischaemia. In this study the drug was not given during 3 hours of reperfusion but nonetheless, infarct size was reduced from 31±6% in untreated controls to 8±2% in the drug-treated group. Auchampach et al (59) have also shown that aprikalim, given intravenously 20 min before and continuing throughout both 90 min ischaemia and 5 h reperfusion, reduced infarct size from 39±4%

to 24±2%. Using similar protocols, Auchampach et al (60) demonstrated that bimakalim reduced infarct size from 46±3% to 32±1% and Grover et al (40) reported that intracoronary pinacidil, given to dogs 10 min before 90 min of regional ischaemia and 5 h of reperfusion, reduced infarct size from 55±7% to 28±5%.

Species Specificity: Do K_{ATP} Channel Openers Limit Infarct Size in all Species?

Owing to the practical difficulties of infarct sizing, most studies of K_{ATP} channel openers and infarct size limitation have been carried out in large mammalian hearts (usually dogs). However, there have been some studies in other species and, in general, these confirm the ability of K_{ATP} channel openers to limit infarct size. Thus, Rohmann et al (61), using pigs subjected to 60 min of regional ischaemia and 120 min of reperfusion, gave bimakalim intravenously starting 15 min before occlusion and continuing for 60 min of reperfusion. Infarct size was reduced by bimakalim from 60±5% to 22±5%. Turning to smaller animals, Toombs et al (62) used rabbits in vivo and administered cromakalim intravenously 30 min before 30 min of regional ischaemia and 2 h of reperfusion; they reported that infarct size was reduced from 47±3% to 33±4%.

Specificity: Is the K_{ATP} Channel Necessarily Involved?

As with the studies of K_{ATP} channel openers and post-ischaemic function, an important question is whether the limitation of infarct size is necessarily achieved by means of a mechanism that involves the K_{ATP} channel. As with the literature on post-ischaemic function, there appears to be strong evidence for a specific involvement of the channel. Thus, Auchampach et al (59) in their dog studies with aprikalim, given 20 min before and throughout 90 min of regional ischaemia and 5 h reperfusion, attenuated the limitation of infarct size by the administration of a bolus of glibenclamide (1 mg/kg) before the ischaemia. Infarct size in the controls was 39±4%, this was reduced to 24±2% in the aprikalim group but was 45±7% in the aprikalim plus glibenclamide group.

When glibenclamide was given alone, it significantly increased infarct size (54±5%) raising the possibility that, with the extended periods of ischaemia used in infarct size studies, some K_{ATP} channels may be open and amenable to blockade.

Timing of Administration: When are the Drugs Active?

As with post-ischaemic function, a number of investigations have been aimed at determining whether K_{ATP} channel openers exert their protective effects before, during or after ischaemia. The results are similar to those found for post-ischaemic function, but the design of some experiments has allowed a more detailed analysis of the times during which the drugs are likely to have their maximum effect. In a study with bimakalim, Auchampach et al (60) administered the drug intravenously either 15 min before the onset of 90 min regional ischaemia and 180 min reperfusion or 5 min before the onset of reperfusion. Whilst pre-ischaemic administration reduced infarct size from 46±3% to 32±1%, pre-reperfusion administration was without effect and resulted in an infarct size of 41±7%. In another dog study, Grover et al (40) compared the effects of intracoronary administration of cromakalim, given 10 min before the onset of ischaemia or 2 min before the onset of reperfusion, in hearts that were subjected to 90 min of regional ischaemia and 5 h of reperfusion. Once again, pre-ischaemic drug administration resulted in a reduction of infarct size from 55±7% to 25±5% whereas administration just before reperfusion was without effect (infarct size being 47±11% vs 46±13%). Whilst the protocols for both of these studies effectively excluded any action of the drug during reperfusion, the results gave no information on whether the drug exerted its beneficial effects before or during ischaemia and, if the latter, when during the period of ischemia the effect is operative. This distinction is of some importance in view of the suggestion (45) that part of the mechanism of action may involve a cardioplegic-like phenomenon in which the drug-induced shortening of action potential hastens mechanical arrest and thereby conserves energy. Some information on this interesting possibility has been provided by several studies by Gross et al (30,31,52,57,63). In one series, they gave either nicorandil or EMD52692 (bimakalim) to dog hearts 10 min *after* the onset of 120 min regional ischaemia and 30 min reperfusion, with the drug infusion continued until the end of the reperfusion period. As shown in Figure 6, after 30 min of reperfusion and despite late administration, significant infarct size limitation was achieved in both instances (38±5% to 19±3% for nicorandil and 45±6% to 20±3% for bimakalim). The magnitude of the reduction was similar to that observed

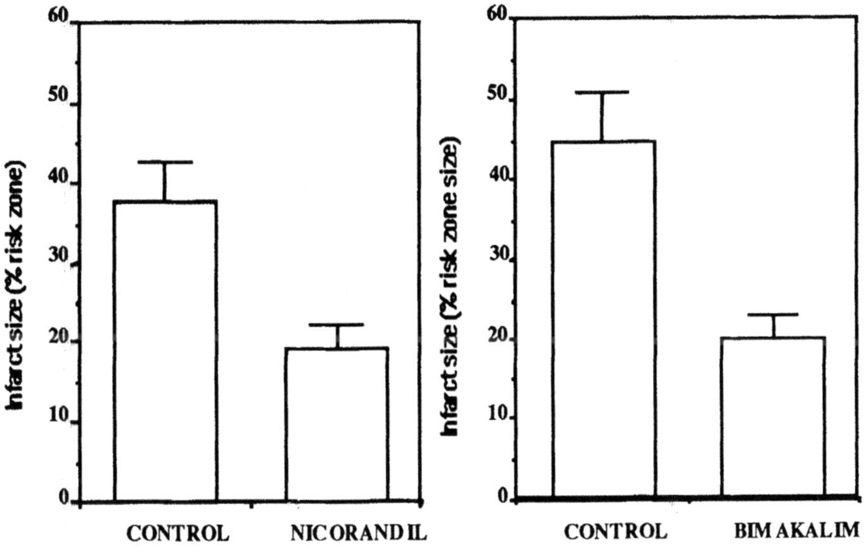

Figure 6: *Delayed administration of K_{ATP} channel blockers and their ability to limit infarct size in the dog heart. When administered to dog hearts 10 min after the onset 120 min of regional ischaemia and 30 min of reperfusion, both bimakalim and nicorandil afforded a similar reduction of infarct size. This figure is based on the work of Gross et al (31).*

in other protocols in which K_{ATP} channel openers were given before ischaemia, an observation that may argue against a cardioplegic-like mechanism of action. However, in another dog-heart study from the same group (63), this time with 60 min of ischaemia and 4 h of reperfusion, 3 doses of bimakalim (0.1, 0.3 or 3.0µg/kg) were given by the intracoronary route for only the first 10 min of ischaemia: infarct size was reduced from its control value of 27±6% to 13±3%, 15±2% and 14±5%, respectively.

Since the relationship between efficacy and time of administration has major clinical logistical implications, there is a clear need for additional studies designed to determine how late into the ischaemic period these drugs can be given without loss of protection and for how long administration is required. In this connection, Endo et al (64) have reported a study in which nicorandil was administered to dog hearts 15 min *after* the onset of a very long period (360 min) of ischaemia and in a protocol that did *not* employ reperfusion, surprisingly (see below), they observed a reduction of infarct size from 93±9% to 64±7%. A large and interesting study has recently been reported by Rohmann et al (61) who used pigs hearts subjected to 60 min of regional ischaemia and 120 min of reperfusion. Bimakalim was given intravenously: (i) for only the 15 min period immediately preceding occlusion (but not during ischaemia or reperfusion), (ii) for 15 min before occlusion and continuously until 60 min of reperfusion and (iii) for 15 min before the onset of reperfusion (i.e., 45 min after the onset of ischaemia) and for the first 60 min of reperfusion. In comparison with untreated controls (in which infarct size was 60±5%) infarct sizes were: 35±7%, 22±5% and 57±4% respectively.

The results of these studies add strength to the suggestion that administration very late into the ischaemic period is less likely to be effective and that, for maximal protection, the drug should be present as close to the time of occlusion as possible. However, this conclusion has been questioned by two recent dog-heart studies: Mizumura et al (58, 65) gave nicorandil or bimakalim intravenously: (i) 15 min before and throughout 60 min of regional ischaemia but not during 3 hours of reperfusion or (ii) 10 min before the end of 60 min of ischaemia and was continued throughout the 3 h of reperfusion. Infarct size in the untreated controls was 31±6%; with nicorandil, this was reduced to 8±2% in the pre-ischaemic treatment group and, surprisingly, to 14±2% in the pre-reperfusion treatment group (the results with bimakalim were similar). Although protection was not as great in the pre-reperfusion group, it was nonetheless present and appears to contradict the findings of other reported studies. One, albeit unlikely, explanation may be that the drug was given 10 min before reperfusion, possibly allowing some anti-ischaemic effects to be manifest, a situation that contrasts with the protocol used by Grover et al (40) who gave the drug only 2 min before reperfusion.

Are All Studies of Infarct Size Limitation Positive?

As with the studies of post-ischaemic functional recovery, a number of negative studies of infarct size question the ability of K_{ATP} channel openers to limit the size of an evolving infarct. Whilst some of these might be dismissed on methodological grounds, others require serious consideration and analysis. Thus, Kitzen et al (66) administered cromakalim and celikalim intravenously to dog hearts starting 10 min before and continuing throughout 90 min of regional ischaemia and 5 h reperfusion. Infarct sizes in the drug-treated groups were 33±13% and 31±10% respectively vs 33±7% in the controls. Kitzen at al (66) also repeated the protocol with the same doses, but this time with the drugs infused by the intracoronary route; they reported that the drugs *increased* infarct size was increased from the control value of 28±6% to 40±6% and 56±6%, respectively. Sakamoto et al (67) reported that pinacidil failed to limit infarct size in dogs; however, this is not surprising in view of the fact that they elected to administer the drug 40 min *after* the onset of ischaemia in a protocol that involved *240 min* of ischaemia before reperfusion was initiated. The negative results reported by Imai et al (68) are of no surprise either since they too gave pinacidil 40 min after the onset of a very long (240 min) period of ischemia. One negative study that is difficult to explain is that reported by Smallwood et al (69) who administered pinacidil or 3-pyridyl pinacidil by the intracoronary route to dog hearts either 10 min before or 10 min after the onset of 90 min of regional ischaemia and 5 h of reperfusion. The drug infusion was continued either until 10 min after the onset of reperfusion or until the end of the experiment. In all four groups, the drugs failed to reduce infarct size. Not only do these results question the ability of pinacidil to limit infarct size but the authors claimed that there was an increase in the incidence or severity of ventricular fibrillation in the drug-treated hearts. Grover et al (40) also reported that pinacidil, when given by the intracoronary route to dog hearts, failed to reduce infarct size. This observation, together with the results of Smallwood et al (69), Imai et al (68) and Sakamoto et al (67), all of whom failed to show protection with pinacidil, raises the possibility that, for some reason, pinacidil is less able to protect against infarction than other drugs in this class. However, as discussed above, Grover et al (40), in the same study, had reported that a higher dose of pinacidil was efficacious.

SUMMARY OF THE EFFECTS OF K_{ATP} CHANNEL OPENERS ON INFARCT SIZE LIMITATION:

Most, but not all, well designed studies demonstrate that all K_{ATP} channel openers, when given *before* ischaemia, can limit infarct size provided reperfusion is instituted within 2 h. If the duration of ischaemia is extended beyond 2 h protection is less likely. However, when protection is observed, it can be attenuated with the K_{ATP} channel blocker glibenclamide. A significant number of studies suggest that protection is possible if the drug is given 10-15 min *after* the onset of ischaemia. How much later the drug can be given whilst still affording protection is not known; if the drug is administered 10 min before reperfusion some protection may be possible but not if it is given immediately before reperfusion (58). All of these results (including some evidence for pro-arrhythmic effects) are fully consistent with the findings of experiments in which post-ischaemic functional recovery was used as an end-point of injury and protection.

MECHANISMS OF CARDIOPROTECTION - QUESTIONING THE CONVENTIONAL VIEW:

A review of the literature quickly reveals that a superficially convincing *conceptual* framework has been developed in an attempt to explain how the manipulation of the K_{ATP} channel influences the evolution of ischaemic injury. As illustrated in Figure 7, central to this framework are the following suppositions or propositions: (i) that ischaemia (like K_{ATP} channel activating drugs) promotes the opening of the K_{ATP} channel, (ii) that K_{ATP} channel openers further facilitate this opening, (iii) that K_{ATP} channel opening increases potassium conductance in myocytes and vascular smooth muscle, (iv) that this causes action potential shortening in myocytes and hyperpolarisation in vascular smooth muscle and that, in both instances, this limits intracellular calcium overload and (v) that this results in vasodilation and reduced contractile performance (or accelerated contractile failure), both of which may afford protection by enhancing coronary flow, reducing cardiac load and conserving ATP. In concert with these effects, it has also been proposed that K_{ATP} channel activation might exert beneficial effects in relation to the utilisation of fatty acids, leucocyte activation, free radical production and prostacyclin metabolism.

However, it is important to stress that much of the above framework is based on: (i) theoretical arguments, (ii) the study of tissues other than the heart, (iii) the use of high (hypotensive) doses that are not clinically relevant and (iii) the potentially dangerous extrapolation of studies with hypoxia to the very different conditions pertaining during ischaemia (this applies particularly to electrophysiological investigations). In the following sections, each of the above propositions is explored and the strength (or otherwise) of supporting evidence assessed.

The Supposition that K_{ATP} Channels Open As a Consequence of Ischaemia:

It is believed that, in normally beating aerobic cardiac tissue, K_{ATP} channels are *closed* and do not contribute to the repolarisation of the myocyte which is mediated by a number of other potassium channels. However (although not essential to the concept that K_{ATP} channel openers are cardioprotective), the concept has been promoted that, during ischaemia (when tissue ATP and pH falls and lactate and adenosine accumulate), some K_{ATP} channels may open and (for the reasons outlined below) protect the heart against ischaemic injury. In this way, ischaemia-induced K_{ATP} channel opening could be viewed as a form of endogenous cardioprotective response (14,20,70,71).

If K_{ATP} channels do open as a consequence of ischaemia and if this does confer endogenous protection on the heart, any intervention that reduces channel opening would be expected to exacerbate ischaemic injury. However, as should be clear from the above review, when models of true ischaemia (as opposed to hypoxia) are employed, relatively little evidence supports the notion that K_{ATP} channel blockers are pro-ischaemic (unless used at high doses (35)). Figure 2 shows clearly that, while glibenclamide can attenuate the protective effects of nicorandil it is without effect if used on its own (32). Such an observation must surely question whether: (i) K_{ATP} channels are necessarily opened as a consequence of myocardial ischaemia and (ii) if open, are as responsive to blockade (44) in the presence of ischaemia.

It should be conceded that some studies (35) do report pro-ischaemic effects when K_{ATP} channel blockers are used on their own. However, if this is true, the clinical consequences of using K_{ATP} channel activators as anti-anginal agents in diabetic patients receiving sulphonylureas should be given careful consideration.

The Supposition that K_{ATP} Channel Activation Shortens Action Potential and Limits Calcium Influx in Myocytes:

Electrophysiological studies suggest that even a relatively small increase in the number of open channels will result in a large outward current (4). It is further argued that this should promote repolarisation and a consequent shortening of action potential duration (not only in contractile tissue but also in conducting tissue such as Purkinje fibres (72)). Although arguments could be mounted to the contrary (W A Coetzee personal communication), shortening of action potential duration in the myocyte would be expected to limit calcium entry through voltage-operated channels (and sodium-calcium exchange) and thus protect the ischaemic tissue.

Yan et al (73) have questioned the role of K_{ATP} channels as mediators of action potential shortening in ischaemia and hypoxia. Certainly, there have been very few studies with true myocardial ischaemia in which K_{ATP} channel-induced protection has been demonstrated whilst, at the same time, substantial or significant changes in action potential duration have been observed (this is especially true when the analysis is limited to studies that employ clinically relevant doses of these drugs). In this connection, in a recent dog-heart study (63) both high and low doses of bimakalim were shown to reduce infarct size to a similar extent despite the fact that the lower dose had *no effect* on action potential duration. Most recently, Grover et al (43) have reported that BMS-180448, a K_{ATP} channel activator devoid of vasodilator properties, is able to improve post-ischaemic contractile function in rats and reduce infarct size in the dog without shortening action potential duration.

The Supposition that K_{ATP} Channel Activation Attenuates Intracellular Calcium Overload and Mechanical Activity:

Another component of the conventional hypothesis is the widely held belief that drug-induced K_{ATP} channel activation limits calcium influx and, as consequence, reduces mechanical function. This in turn is supposed to hasten contractile arrest, thereby conserving ATP for tissue protection (74). However, no *direct* evidence is available for such a drug-induced reduction in calcium overload and little evidence from ischaemic preparations to support the notion that the time-to-mechanical arrest is substantially shortened.

The Supposition that K_{ATP} Channel Activation Improves Flow to Ischaemic Tissue:

In addition to their effects on the myocyte, K_{ATP} channel openers would, it has been argued, be expected to influence vascular smooth muscle, possibly at concentrations lower than those required for the activation of myocyte channels (17). The primary action of these drugs on vascular smooth muscle is to hyperpolarise the resting membrane potential (1). This may possibly limit calcium influx through voltage-operated channels which, in turn, will promote vasodilatation and possibly also combat coronary spasm (13). Whilst K_{ATP} channel activation can undoubtedly promote vasodilation in a number of isolated vascular preparations, it is far from clear whether this translates to improved nutritive flow to an ischaemic zone in a whole heart. Several important areas are in need of clarification including: (i) the precise level in the vascular tree at which these drugs act (this is likely to be at the level of the resistance vessels), (ii) although unlikely (13), it is not clear whether, under any circumstances, they might precipitate a steal phenomenon, (iii) whether the ischaemia alone is sufficient to ensure maximal vasodilation of stenotic vessels and (iv) whether collateral vessels, if they exist, are responsive to these agents. If K_{ATP} channel openers can exert such beneficial effects, they would be expected to protect the heart by a direct reduction in the severity of ischaemia. This might be particularly important in the case of nicorandil, with its unique secondary nitrate property, in which additional benefit might also be expected through a direct effect on vascular smooth muscle leading to dilation of large vessels (75). However, one might question the importance of such a component mechanism on the ground that these drugs afford excellent protection in: (i) zero flow, globally ischaemic preparations in which there is no scope for vasodilation and (ii) in rat and pig hearts that possess few, if any, collateral vessels.

A vascular basis to the protective mechanisms of K_{ATP} channel openers could, of course, involve peripheral vasodilation and consequent unloading of the heart. However, if such mechanism were central to the protective properties of these drugs it is difficult to see how they could be so protective in isolated perfused-heart preparations in which peripheral factors are totally excluded. An additional argument against vasodilation as a major component of the cardioprotective action of K_{ATP} channel openers comes from the recent study by Grover et al (43) who showed that BMS-180448, an agent devoid of vasodilator properties, could reduce infarct size and improve post-ischaemic recovery to an extent comparable to that achieved with other K_{ATP} channel openers.

The Supposition that K_{ATP} Channel Openers Exhibit Selectivity for Ischaemic Tissue:

It is questionable whether, in aerobic tissue in the *absence* of ischaemia, clinically relevant doses of K_{ATP} channel opening drugs have sufficient potency to promote channel opening. However, an attractive component of the conventional K_{ATP} cardioprotection hypothesis is that, *during ischaemia,* there exists a synergistic effect between the drug and the ischaemia such that the probability of channel opening is greatly enhanced. From this it follows that, at moderate doses, these drugs might exhibit selectivity for ischaemic tissue by failing to act on non-ischaemic or peripheral tissue whilst (as a consequence of reduced tissue pH and ATP content which allows K_{ATP} channel activation at lower drug concentrations) preferentially acting on tissue that is ischaemic. Indeed, it could be argued that, the more ischaemic the tissue, the greater the potency of these drugs. As attractive as this hypothesis is, there is no direct evidence to support it in models of ischaemia in whole hearts.

The Proposition of Other Mechanisms?

The concerns outlined above serve to highlight increasing doubt over the mechanisms of action of a very powerful group of drugs. Whilst this in no way diminishes the potential for such drugs to exert major therapeutic effects, it does point to the pressing need for more carefully designed and relevant experiment work. Uncertainty over the mechanisms of action has led some investigators to consider alternative ways in which protection may be achieved. These include the possibilities that K_{ATP} channel openers may influence: (i) intracellular calcium control mechanisms (1,49), possibly through mitochondrial K_{ATP} channels (17,76), (ii) neutrophil function (an action that is unlikely to be important in isolated-heart preparations) and free radical production (30,77), (iii) fatty acid metabolism (30,78) and (iv) prostacyclin production (30). However, none of these are supported unequivocally by available data and none is likely to be able to account for the striking protection seen under so many different conditions and in so many studies.

One area of topical interest is preconditioning and the possibility that this protective phenomenon may involve adenosine A_1 receptor-mediated activation of the K_{ATP} channel. As a consequence, it has been suggested that K_{ATP} channel activation may be able to mimic preconditioning. Since this is the subject of another chapter in this book(see chapter by Gross & Yellon reviews, no attempt will be made to cover it here.

THE ADDED COMPLICATION OF K_{ATP} CHANNELS AND ARRHYTHMIAS:

Whilst there are strong arguments that K_{ATP} channel openers should protect the myocyte and the vasculature against acute ischaemic injury, arguments can also be advanced that potassium channel openers might, at the same time, be detrimental because they may be pro-arrhythmic (Figure 7). On the other hand, arguments have also been advanced that K_{ATP} channel openers may be anti-arrhythmic (for reviews of these opposing views see (19,72,81-87), particularly under conditions where acute ischemia is not involved. Although extensively discussed, and although there have been many cellular and sub-cellular studies of the electrophysiological consequences of K_{ATP} channel modulation, relatively few prospective, in vivo, experimental studies have been carried out of the effects of K_{ATP} channel modulation on electrical stability in whole hearts with either regional or global ischaemia. Furthermore, of those studies that have been reported, few, if any, have: (i) used adequate animal numbers, (ii) employed clinically relevant doses or (iii) controlled fully for critically important determinants of arrhythmogenesis such as heart rate, autonomic tone, collateral flow and the size of the risk zone.

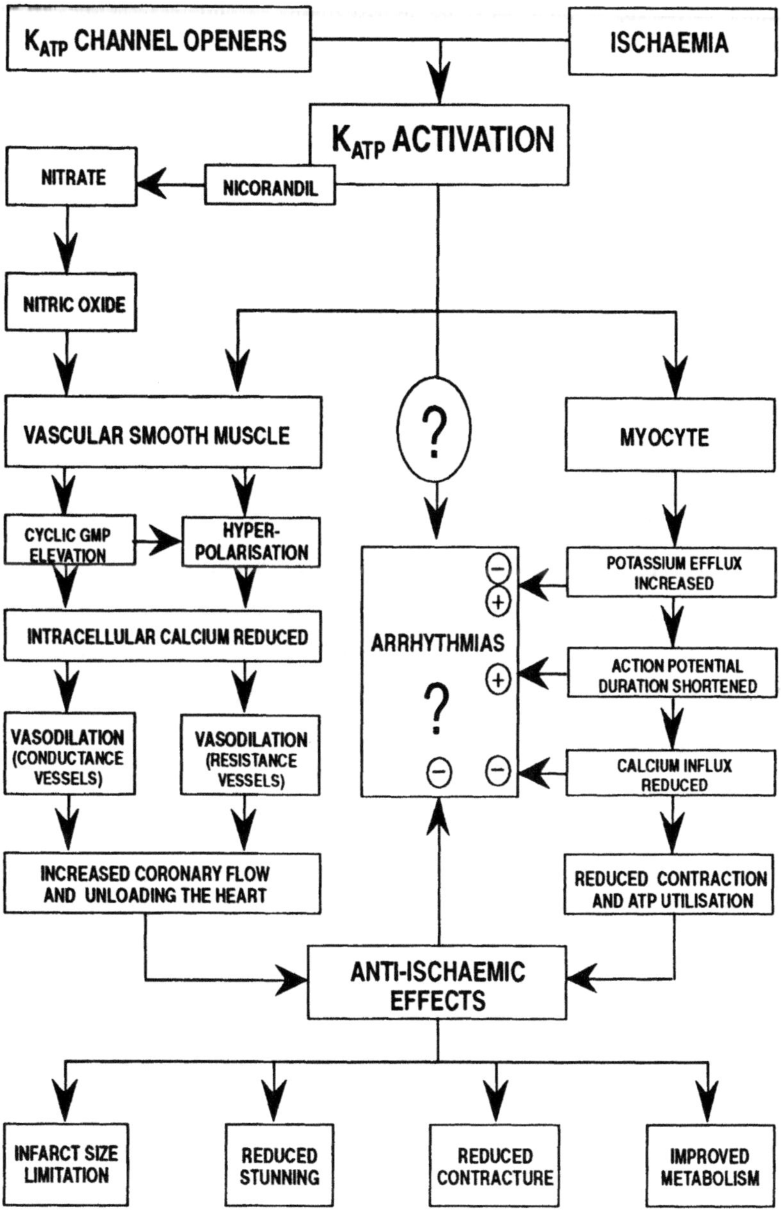

Figure 7: *Diagrammatic illustration of the conventional view on the way in which K_{ATP} channel activation, either by ischaemia or channel opening drugs, influences vascular smooth muscle and myocytes so as to exert an anti-ischaemic effect. The controversial consequences of these changes on susceptibility to arrhythmias is also indicate.*

Despite the paucity of prospective controlled studies, a number of studies (usually with infarct size or post-ischaemic contractile function as primary end-points) have noted the effects on susceptibility to arrhythmias. In the setting of acute myocardial ischaemia most (but not all) such studies suggest that K_{ATP} channel openers have a tendency to be pro-fibrillatory (88,89), particularly when the drugs are used at high (hypotensive) doses. By contrast, most studies with K_{ATP} channel blockers indicate that these drugs tend to be anti-arrhythmic.

On theoretical grounds, any pro-arrhythmic effect of K_{ATP} channel openers would be expected to stem from their ability to increase potassium conductance and decrease refractory period by shortening action potential duration. If this were to occur preferentially in a zone of regional ischaemia, then K_{ATP} channel openers would be expected to *amplify* any ischaemia-induced heterogeneity of potassium accumulation and action potential shortening and thereby increase the susceptibility to arrhythmias. As discussed by Billman et al (83), inhomogeneities of potassium conductance and accumulation (such as occur either between normal and ischaemic tissue during regional ischaemia or arise *within* an ischaemic zone due to transmural gradients of ischaemia) will result in regional differences in repolarisation and action potential duration. As a consequence, spatial heterogeneities (dispersion) of the refractory period may predispose to fragmentation of impulse conduction, re-entry and ventricular fibrillation or ventricular tachycardia. In support of this, drugs that *widen* action potential duration in an ischaemic zone generally possess anti-arrhythmic effects. If K_{ATP} channel openers tend to shorten action potential duration in ischaemic tissue then they might also be expected to increase injury currents between ischaemic and non-ischaemic tissue and thus promote ectopic activity.

Countering the preceding arguments, and as discussed above, there is growing doubt over whether, or to what extent, K_{ATP} channel openers actually shorten action potential duration in models of true ischaemia, especially when used at clinically relevant doses (63). If this turns out to be the case, then many of the theoretical arguments for a pro-arrhythmic effect of these drugs disappear. This might even serve to strengthen theoretical arguments for an *anti*-arrhythmic property of K_{ATP} channel openers. Such arguments would be made much easier if these drugs preferentially shortened action potential in *non*-ischaemic tissue, however, as discussed above, this is very unlikely to occur. There are several arguments that may be advanced in support of an anti-arrhythmic effect of K_{ATP} channel opening. Thus, according to the classical view, an area of slow conduction is required for re-entry, whilst activation K_{ATP} channels may initially decrease action potential duration (a pro-arrhythmic mechanism) it might also prevent the generation of action potentials in an area of slow conduction and thus create bi-directional conduction block (an anti-arrhythmic mechanism). Another argument (again dependent upon channel opening in non-ischaemic tissue) relates to the possibility that these drugs might reduce regional gradients in extracellular potassium, however, not only is it questionable whether the drugs act on normal tissue but, if they did, only small amounts of potassium would be released and these would be expected to be washed away by normal blood flow.

One plausible argument for an anti-arrhythmic effect of K_{ATP} channel activation relates to the fact that there is a relationship between the severity of ischaemia and the severity (or time-to-onset) of resulting arrhythmias. Any intervention, such a K_{ATP} channel opener, that reduces ischaemic injury (by conserving ATP or increasing flow) might reasonably be expected to protect the heart against arrhythmias.

The arrhythmogenic potential of K_{ATP} channel activation remains a complex and controversial issue. It is clear, that predicting the effects of K_{ATP} channel activators on susceptibility to arrhythmias is critically dependent upon a clear understanding of the relative effects of these drugs on action potential duration in both ischaemic and normal tissue. This information is not yet available and until it is, it becomes very difficult to convincingly explain how K_{ATP} channel openers could be anti-arrhythmic in conditions such as regional ischaemia. As discussed by Wilde (72,81) and others (17,90), the pro-arrhythmic properties of K_{ATP} channel openers can certainly be disputed, the phenomenon is undoubtedly species-dependent, dose-dependent and model-dependent. It may also be drug-dependent and will certainly depend on the cardiac pathology (stable vs unstable angina vs evolving infarction vs established infarction), the type of arrhythmia and its underlying mechanism (72). Thus, although K_{ATP} channel activation may increase susceptibility to arrhythmias that are caused by re-entry, those arising as a consequence of abnormal automaticity or triggered activity might be expected to be reduced by K_{ATP} channel activation. The balance of these complex and sometimes conflicting effects is controversial (86,87,91-94), and clearly in need of detailed prospective investigations in which the relative pro- and anti-arrhythmic risks are assessed and compared to the benefit of the anti-ischemic properties of these drugs. However, in assessing overall clinical risk benefit profile, it is perhaps worth noting that, to date, extensive clinical experience with K_{ATP} channel openers (used either as anti-hypertensive or anti-anginal agents) have not uncovered any serious pro-arrhythmic effects and therefore the potential problems may well have been overestimated (72).

GENERAL CONCLUSIONS:

Activators of the ATP-sensitive potassium channel undoubtedly possess anti-ischaemic properties that allow them to *slow the rate* of development of ischaemic injury such that, upon reperfusion after a fixed ischaemic insult, infarct size is smaller and/or post-ischaemic functional recovery is improved. Although not discussed here, this conclusion is supported by the results of other studies that used other end-points (e.g. contracture, metabolism or enzyme leakage) of injury and protection. Whilst K_{ATP} channel openers are undoubtedly anti-ischaemic it does not necessarily follow that K_{ATP} channel blockers are pro-ischaemic. There is some [59], but relatively little, evidence that they are able to exacerbate either post-ischaemic contractile dysfunction or increase infarct size. This raises the question as to whether K_{ATP} channels are necessarily open during unmodified ischaemia.

A number of studies report data to suggest that K_{ATP} channel blockers can exert anti-arrhythmic effects and that K_{ATP} channel openers may, under certain conditions be pro-arrhythmic. However, these potentially deleterious effects may be species-dependent, model-dependent and dose-dependent and their clinical risk may have been overestimated.

The ability of K_{ATP} channel blockers to attenuate the ability of K_{ATP} channels openers to reduce infarct size, improve post-ischaemic function or promote arrhythmias provides compelling evidence to support the notion that the drugs act through a specific K_{ATP} channel-dependent mechanism. The nature of this mechanism, which appears to operate primarily during the ischaemic period, remains to be resolved as does the balance of benefit derived from the actions of these drugs on the myocyte and the vascular smooth muscle. This applies particularly to nicorandil with is unique nitrate property, which is capable of promoting vasodilatation by a direct nitric oxide-mediated mechanism that is independent of the effect of the drug on K_{ATP} channel-mediated vasodilation. The remarkable similarity in findings between the studies of 'stunning' and infarct size lend support to the suggestion that a substantial degree of the observed protection is likely to occur at the level of the myocardium, without the requirement for an involvement of peripheral vasodilation, innervation or blood-borne factors such as leucocytes.

In conclusion, K_{ATP} channel opening drugs represent a new class of drugs that may offer exciting new therapeutic opportunities under conditions in which a reduction in the severity and consequences of an episode of ischaemia is desirable. Possible clinical applications include various forms of angina, myocardial infarction with early thrombolysis and cardiac surgery instances in which the prognosis may be affected by the consequences of stunning or infarction. Clearly, this family of drugs is worthy of further investigations aimed at resolving a number of important, but as yet unanswered, questions.

REFERENCES:

1. Quast U: Do the K^+ channel openers relax smooth muscle by opening K^+ channels? TIPS 1993;14:332-337.
2. Cook NS: The pharmacology of potassium channels and their therapeutic potential. TIPS 1988;9:21-28.
3. Longman SD, Hamilton TC: Potassium channel activator drugs: mechanism of action, pharmacological proterties, and therapeutic potential. Med Res Rev 1992;12:73-148.
4. Findlay I, Faivre J-F: ATP-sensitive K channels in heart muscle. Spare channels.FEBS 1991;279:95-97.
5. Weston AH, Edwards G: Recent progress in potassium channel opener pharmacology. Biochem Pharmacol 1992;43:47-54.
6. Nichols CG, Lederer WJ: Adenosine triphosphate-sensitive potassium channels in the cardiovascular system. Am J Physiol 1991;261:H1675-H1686.
7. Coetzee WA: ATP-sensitive potassium channels and myocardial ischemia: why do they open? Cardiovasc Drugs Ther 1992;6:201-208.
8. Richer C, Pratz J, Mulder P, et al: Cardiovascular and biological effects of K^+ channel openers, vasorelaxant and cardioprotective properties. Life Sci 1990;47:1693-1705.
9. Cook NS, Quast U: Potassium channel pharmacology, in Cook NS (ed): Potassium channels, structures, classification, function and therapeutic potential. Chichester, Ellis Horwood, 1990, pp 181-255.
10. Ashcroft SJH, Ashcroft FM: Properties and functions of ATP-sensitive K^+ channels. Cell Sig 1990;2:197-214.
11. Edwards G, Weston AH: The pharmacology of ATP-sensitive potassium channels. Ann Rev Pharmacol Toxicol 1993;33:597-637.
12. De Weille JR: Modulation of ATP sensitive potassium channels. Cardiovasc Res 1992;26:1017-1020.
13. Sakai K: Nicorandil: animal pharmacology. Am J Cardiol 1989;63:2J-10J.

14. Cavero I, Djellas Y, Guillon J-M: Ischemic myocardial cell protection conferred by the opening of ATP-sensitive potassium channels. Cardiovasc Drugs Ther 1995;9:245-255.

15. Lazdunski M: Potassium channels: structure-function relationships, diversity, and pharmacology. Cardiovasc Drugs Ther 1992;6:313-319.

16. Lazdunski M: ATP-sensitive potassium channels: an overview. J Cardiovasc Pharmacol 1994;24 (Suppl.4):S1-S5.

17. Grover GJ: Protective effects of ATP sensitive potassium channel openers in models of myocardial ischaemia. Cardiovasc Res 1994;28:778-782.

18. Cavero I, Premmereur J: ATP sensitive potassium channel openers are of potential benefit in ischaemic heart disease. Cardiovasc Res 1994;28:32-33.

19. Opie LH: Modulation of ischemia by regulation of the ATP-sensitive potassium channel. Cardiovasc Drugs Ther 1993;7:507-513.

20. Cole WC: ATP-sensitive K^+ channels in cardiac ischemia: an endogenous mechanism for protection of the heart. Cardiovasc Drugs Ther 1993;7 (Suppl.3):527-537.

21. Gross GJ, Auchampach JA: Role of ATP dependent potassium channels in myocardial ischaemia. Cardiovasc Res 1992;26:1011-1016.

22. Siegl P: Blockers of ATP sensitive potassium current are of potential benefit in ischaemic heart disease. Cardiovasc Res 1994;28:31-33.

23. Hearse DJ, Yellon DM: Why are we still in doubt about infarct size limitation? The experimentalist's viewpoint, in Hearse DJ, Yellon DM (eds): Therapeutic approaches to infarct size limitation. New York, Raven Press, 1984, pp 17-41.

24. Hearse DJ: The protection of the ischemic myocardium: surgical success versus clinical failure. Prog Cardiovasc Dis 1988;6:381-402.

25. Hearse DJ, Bolli R: Reperfusion-induced injury: manifestation, mechanisms and clinical relevance. Trends Cardiovasc Med 1991;1:233-240.

26. Grover GJ, Sleph PG, Parham CS: Nicorandil improves postischemic contractile function independently of direct myocardial effects. J Cardiovasc Pharmacol 1990;15:698-705.

27. D'Alonzo AJ, Darbenzio RB, Parham CS, et al: Effects of intracoronary cromakalim on postischaemic contractile function and action potential duration. Cardiovasc Res 1992;26:1046-1053.

28. Gross GJ, Warltier DC, Hardman HF: Comparative effects of nicorandil, a nicotinamide nitrate derivative, and nifedipine on myocardial reperfusion injury in dogs. J Cardiovasc Pharmacol 1987;10:535-542.

29. Gross GJ, Pieper GM, Warltier DC: Comparative effects of nicorandil, nitroglycerin, nicotinic acid, and SG-86 on the metabolic status and functional recovery of the ischemic-reperfused myocardium. J Cardiovasc Pharmacol 1987;10 (Suppl.8):S76-S84.

30. Gross G, Pieper G, Farber NE, et al: Effects of nicorandil on coronary circulation and myocardial ischemia. Am J Cardiol 1989;63:11J-17J.

31. Gross GJ, Auchampach JA, Maruyama M, et al: Cardioprotective effects of nicorandil. J Cardiovasc Pharmacol 1992;20 (Suppl.3):S22-S28.

32. Auchampach JA, Cavero I, Gross GJ: Nicorandil attenuates myocardial dysfunction associated with transient ischemia by opening ATP-dependent potassium channels. J Cardiovasc Pharmacol 1992;20:765-771.

33. Auchampach JA, Maruyama M, Cavero I, et al: Pharmacological evidence for a role of ATP-dependent potassium channels in myocardial stunning. Circulation 1992;86:311-319.

34. Udvary E, Szilvassy Z, Papp JG: Glibenclamide reverses cromakalim-induced anti-ischemic effect in conscious rabbits.
Pharmacol Res 1992;25 (Suppl.2):179-180.

35. Cole WC, McPherson CD, Sontag D: ATP-regulated K^+ channels protect the myocardium against ischemia/reperfusion damage. Circ Res 1991;69:571-581.

36. Grover GJ, Sleph PG, Dzwonczyk S: Pharmacologic profile of cromakalim in the treatment of myocardial ischemia in isolated rat hearts and anesthetized dogs. J Cardiovasc Pharmacol 1990;16:853-864.

37. McCullough JR, Normandin DE, Conder ML, et al: Specific block of the anti-ischemic actions of cromakalim by sodium 5-hydroxydecanoate. Circ Res 1991;69:949-958.

38. Sargent CA, Smith MA, Dzwonczyk S, et al: Effect of potasium channel blockade on the anti-ischemic actions of mechanistically diverse agents. J Pharmacol Exp Ther 1991;259:97-103.

39. Grover GJ, Dzwonczyk S, Sleph PG: Reduction of ischemic damage in isolated rat hearts by the potassium channel opener, RP 52891. Eur J Pharmacol 1990;191:11-18.

40. Grover GJ, Dzwonczyk S, Parham CS, et al: The protective effects of cromakalim and pinacidil on reperfusion function and infarct size in isolated perfused rat hearts and anesthetized dogs. Cardiovasc Drugs Ther 1990;4:465-474.

41. Grover GJ, Newburger J, Sleph PG, et al: Cardioprotective effects of the potassium channel opener cromakalim: stereoselectivity and effects on myocardial adenine nucleotides. J Pharmacol Exp Ther 1991;257:156-162.

42. Grover GJ, McCullough JR, Henry EE, et al: Anti-ischemic effects of the potasium channel activators pinacidil and cromakalim and the reversal of these effects with the potassium channel blocker glyburide. J Pharmacol Exp Ther 1989;251:98-104.

43. Grover GJ, McCullough JR, D'Alonzo AJ, et al: Cardioprotective profile of the cardiac-selective ATP-sensitive potassium channel opener BMS-180448. J Cardiovasc Pharmacol 1995;25:40-50.

44. Findlay I: Sulphonylurea drugs no longer inhibit ATP-sensitive K^+ channels during metabolic stress in cardiac muscle. J Pharmacol Exp Ther 1993;266:456-467.

45. Galiñanes M, Shattock MJ, Hearse DJ: Effects of potassium channel modulation during global ischaemia in isolated rat heart with and without cardioplegia. Cardiovasc Res 1992;26:1063-1068.

46. Irie H: Experimental studies on ischemic injury and reperfusion injury to the cardiac sarcoplasmic reticulum. The myocardial protective effect of nicorandil. Jap Circ J 1988;52:563-569.

47. Sugimoto S, Puddu PE, Monti F, et al: Pretreatment with the adenosine triphosphate-sensitive potasium channel opener nicorandil and improved myocardial protection during high-potassium cardioplegic hypoxia. J Thorac Cardiovasc Surg 1994;108:455-466.

48. Cohen NM, Wise RM, Wechsler AS, et al: Elective cardiac arrest with hyperpolarizing adenosine triphosphate-sensitive potassium channel opener. A novel form of myocardial protection?
J Thorac Cardiovasc Surg 1993;106:317-328.

49. Grover GJ: Protective effects of ATP-sensitive potassium-channel openers in experimental myocardial ischemia. J Cardiovasc Pharmacol 1994;24 (Suppl.4):S18-S27.

50. Ohta H, Jinno Y, Harada K, et al: Cardioprotective effects of KRN2391 and nicorandil on ischemic dysfunction in perfused rat heart. Eur J Pharmacol 1991;204:171-177.

51. Mitani A, Konoshita K, Fukamachi K, et al: Effects of glibenclamide and nicorandil on cardiac function during ischemia and reperfusion in isolated perfused rat hearts. Am J Physiol 1991;261:H1864-H1871.

52. Haneda T, Ichihara K, Onodera S: Effects of nicorandil and nipradilol on ischemic myocardium in perfused rat heart. Eur J Pharmacol 1989;162:81-87.

53. Pieper GM, Gross GJ: Protective effect of nicorandil on postischemic function and tissue adenine nucleotides following a brief period of low-flow global ischemia in the isolated perfused rat heart. Pharmacology 1989;38:205-213.

54. Qiu Y, Galiñanes M, Hearse DJ: Protective effect of nicorandil as an additive to continuous warm cardioplegia. J Thorac Cardiovasc Surg 1995;(in press)

55. Rees SA, Curtis MJ: A pharmacological analysis in rat of the role of the ATP-sensitive potassium channel as target for antifibrillatory intervention in acute myocardial ischemia. J Cardiovasc Pharmacol 1995;(in press)

56. Gross GJ, Auchampach JA: Blockade of ATP-sensitive potassium channels prevents myocardial preconditioning in dogs. Circ Res 1992;70:223-233.

57. Lamping KA, Christensen CW, Pelc LR, et al: Effects of nicorandil and nifedipine on protection of ischemic myocardium. J Cardiovasc Pharmacol 1984;6:536-542.

58. Mizumura T, Nithipatikom K, Gross GJ: Effects of nicorandil and glyceryl trinitrate on infarct size, adenosine release, and neutrophil infiltration in the dog. Cardiovasc Res 1995;29:482-489.

59. Auchampach JA, Maruyama M, Cavero I, et al: The new K^+ channel opener aprikalim (RP 52891) reduces experimental infarct size in dogs in the absence of hemodynamic changes. J Pharmacol Exp Ther 1991;259:961-967.

60. Auchampach JA, Gross GJ: Reduction in myocardial infarct size by the new potassium channel opener bimakalim. J Cardiovasc Pharmacol 1994;23:554-561.

61. Rohmann S, Weygandt H, Schelling P, et al: Effects of bimakalim (EMD 52692), on opener of ATP sensitive potassium channels, on infarct size, coronary blood flow, regional wall function, and oxygen consumption in swine. Cardiovasc Res 1994;28:858-863.

62. Toombs CF, Norman NR, Groppi VE, et al: Limitation of myocardial injury with the potassium channel opener cromakalim and the nonvasoactive analog U-89,232: vascular vs. cardiac actions in vitro and in vivo. J Pharmacol Exp Ther 1992;263:1261-1268.

63. Yao Z, Gross GJ: Effects of the KATP channel opener bimakalim on coronary blood flow, monophasic action potential duration, and infarct size in dogs. Circulation 1994;89:1769 1775.

64. Endo T, Nejima J, Kiuchi K, et al: Reduction of size of myocardial infarction with nicorandil, a new antianginal drug, after coronary artery occlusion in dogs. J Cardiovasc Pharmacol 1988;12:587-592.

65. Mizumura T, Kithipatikom K, Gross GJ: Bimakalim, an ATP-sensitive potassium channel opener, mimics the effects of ischemic preconditioning to reduce infarct size, adenosine release and neutrophil function in dogs. Circulation 1995;(in press)

66. Kitzen JM, McCallum JD, Harvey C, et al: Potassium channel activators cromakalim and celikalim (WAY-120,491) fail to decrease myocardial infarct size in the anesthetized canine. Pharmacology 1992;45:71-82.

67. Sakamoto S, Liang C, Stone CK, et al: Effects of pinacidil on myocardial blood flow and infarct size after acute left anterior descending coronary artery occlusion and reperfusion in awake dogs with and without a coexisting left circumflex coronary artery stenosis. J Cardiovasc Pharmacol 1989;14:747-755.

68. Iami N, Liang C-S, Stone CK, et al: Comparative effects of nitroprusside and pinacidil on myocardial blood flow and infarct size in awake dogs with acute myocardial infarction. Circulation 1988;77:705-711.

69. Smallwood JK, Schelm JA, Bemis KG, et al: Effect of activation of ATP-dependent potassium channels with (-)-Pinacidil and (-)-3-3pyridyl pinacidil on infarct size in a canine model of ischemia-reperfusion injury. J Cardiovasc Pharmacol 1993;22:731-743.

70. Escande D, Cavero I: K^+ channel openers and 'natural' cardioprotection. TIPS 1992;13:269-272.

71. Yao Z, Gross GJ: Protective effects of ATP-sensitive potassium channel: an endogenous cardioprotective mechanism. J Cardiovasc Pharmacol 1994;24 (Suppl.4):28-34.

72. Wilde AAM, Janse MJ: Electrophysiological effects of ATP sensitive potassium channel modulation: implications for arrhythmogenesis. Cardiovasc Res 1994;28:16-24.

73. Yan G-X, Yamada KA, Kleber AG, et al: Dissociation between cellular K^+ loss, reduction in repolarization time, and tissue ATP levels during myocardial hypoxia and ischemia. Circulation Research 1993;72:560-570.

74. McPherson CD, Pierce GN, Cole WC: Ischemic cardioprotection by ATP-sensitive K^+ channels involves high-energy phosphate preservation. Am J Physiol 1993;265:H1809-H1818.

75. Bolotina VM, Najibi S, Palacino JJ, et al: Nitric oxide directly activates calcium-denpendent potassium channels in vascular smooth muscle. Nature 1994;368:850-853.

76. Inoue I, Nagase H, Kishi K, et al: ATP-sensitive K^+ channel in the mitochondrial inner membrane. Nature 1991;352:244-247.

77. Pieper GM, Gross GJ: Anti-free-radical and neutrophil-modulating properties of the nitrovasodilator, nicorandil. Cardiovasc Drugs Ther 1992;6:225-232.

78. Pieper GM, Gross GJ: Salutary action of nicorandil, a new antianginal drug, on myocardial metabolism during ischemia and on postischemic function in a canine preparation of brief, repetitive coronary artery occlusions: comparison with isosorbide dinitrate. Circulation 1987;76:916-928.

79. Gross GJ, Yao Z, Auchampach JA: Role of ATP-sensitive potassium channels in ischemic preconditioning, in Przyklenk K, Kloner RA, Yellon DM (eds): Ischemic preconditioning: the concept of endogenous cardioprotection. Kluwer Academic Publishers, 1994, pp 125-135.

80. Parratt JR, Kane KA: K_{ATP} channels in ischaemic preconditioning. Cardiovasc Res 1994;28:783-787.

81. Wilde AAM: K_{ATP}-channel opening and arrhythmogenesis. J Cardiovasc Pharmacol 1994;24 (Suppl.4):S35-S40.

82. Colatsky TJ, Follmer CH: K^+ channel blockers and activators in cardiac arrhythmias. Cardiovasc Drug Rev 1989;7:199-109.

83. Billman GE: Role of ATP sensitive potassium channel in extracellular potassium accumulation and cardiac arrhythmias during myocardial ischaemia. Cardiovasc Res 1994;28:762-769.

84. Coronel R: Heterogeneity in extracellular potassium concentration during early myocardial ischaemia and reperfusion: implications for arrhythmogenesis. Cardiovasc Res 1994;28:770-777.

85. D'Alonzo AJ, Dabenzio RB, Hess TA, et al: Effect of potassium on the action of the K_{ATP} modulators cromakalim, pinacidil, or glibenclamide on arrhythmias in isolated perfused rat heart subjected to regional ischaemia. Cardiovasc Res 1994;28:881-887.

86. Baghdady R, Nichols C: Letter to the Editor. Cardiovasc Res 1994;28:135-136.

87. Chi L, Black SC, Friedrichs GS, et al: Letter to the Editor. Cardiovasc Res 1994;28:136-137.

88. Wollenben CD, Sanguinetti MC, Siegl PKS: Influence of ATP-sensitive potassium channel modulators on ischemia-induced fibrillation in isolated rat hearts. J Mol Cell Cardiol 1989;21:783-788.

89. Chi L, Uprichard AC, Lucchesi BR: Profibrillatory actions of pinacidil in a conscious canine model of sudden coronary death. J Cardiovasc Pharmacol 1990;15:452-464.
90. Di Diego JM, Antzelevitch C: Pinacidil-induced electrical heterogeneity and extrasystolic activity in canine ventricular tissues. Does activation of ATP-regulated protassium current promote phase 2 reentry? Circulation 1993;88:1177-1189.
91. Black SC, Lucchesi BR: Potassium channels are likely to be proarrhythmic in the diseased human heart. Cardiovasc Res 1994;28:923-924.
92. D'Alonzo AJ, Grover GJ: Potassium channel openers are unlikely to be proarrhythmic in the diseased human heart. Cardiovasc Res 1994;28:924-925.
93. Billman G: Letter to the Editor. Cardiovasc Res 1994;28:137-138.
94. Gross G: Letter to the Editor. Cardiovasc Res 1994;28:139-140.

4

THE RELATIONSHIP BETWEEN THE K_{ATP} CHANNEL AND MYOCARDIAL PRECONDITIONING

GARRET J GROSS* and DEREK M YELLON
*Department of Pharmacology & Toxicology,Medical College of Wisconsin
8701 Watertown Plank Road,Milwaukee, USA and
The Hatter Institute, Department of Academic & Clinical Cardiology, University College London Medical School, & Hospital, Grafton Way, London WC1E 6DB. UK.

INTRODUCTION

The Role of the ATP-sensitive potassium channel (K_{ATP}) in Myocardial Ischemia:
Since the original discovery of the K_{ATP} channel by Noma (1) in 1983, numerous studies have been performed in whole cells and membrane patches to determine the factors which regulate its activity in the heart, and in addition to ATP, a number of endogenous modulators of K_{ATP} channel activity have been identified. These include adenosine, the ADP/ATP ratio, certain nucleotide diphosphates, Mg^{++}, pH, lactate and protein kinase C (2,3).
The physiological and pathophysiological function of this channel in the heart has also been a subject of intense interest and Noma (1) originally proposed that this channel might serve an endogenous cardioprotective role by the mechanisms depicted in Figure 1. The major electrophysiological effect observed in cardiac myocytes as a result of K_{ATP} channel opening during ischemia is a rapid decrease in the ventricular action potential duration. This effect has been shown to result in a rapid loss of electrical and mechanical activity and a reduction in calcium entry or overload via voltage-operated calcium channels and Na-Ca exchange (4). All these effects would be expected to produce a marked reduction in myocardial oxygen consumption, preserve cellular energy stores and delay cell injury or death if timely restoration of blood flow were to occur.

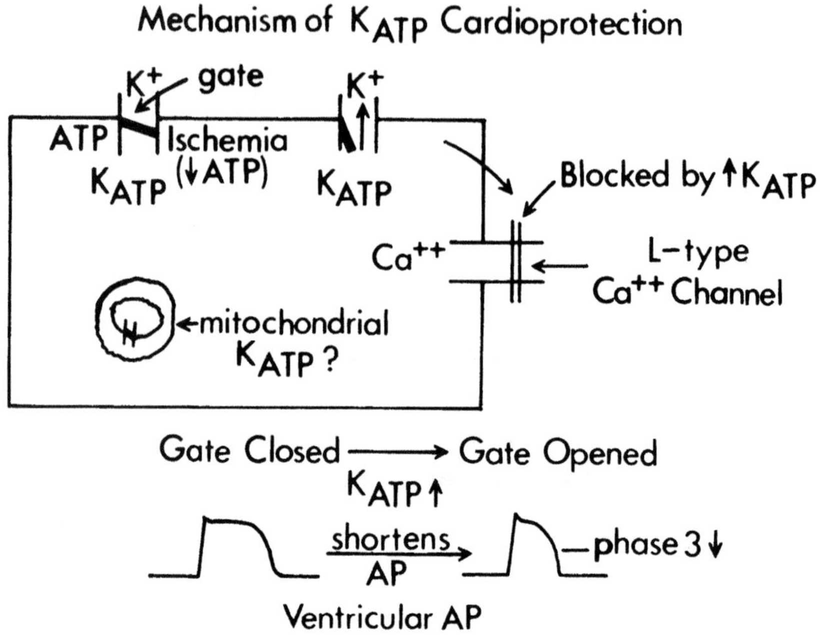

Figure 1. A schematic diagram illustrating the major mechanism and the consequences of opening the ATP-sensitive potassium channel (K_{ATP}) during ischemia, hypoxia or metabolic inhibition [1]. Activation of the K_{ATP} channel produces a decrease in action potential duration in cardiac myocytes by enhancing phase 3 repolarization. This action reduces calcium entry via L-type calcium channels and produces membrane hyperpolarization particularly in vascular smooth muscle. These electrophysiological effects lead to a rapid loss in cellular, electrical and mechanical function, a reduction in calcium overload, a preservation of cellular energy stores, a reduction in cell swelling (perhaps due to a recently discovered mitochondrial K_{ATP} channel) and an increase in coronary blood flow. All of these actions would delay cell death and result in a decrease in myocardial infarct size if timely reperfusion were to occur.

Indeed, a number of studies, including many performed in Gross' laboratory, indicate that K_{ATP} channel opening is cardioprotective (5,6,7) and the results concerning the beneficial effects of K_{ATP} channel openers in myocardial stunning and infarction have been described in detail in the preceding chapter by Hearse. In addition to these studies with K_{ATP} openers, it has also been shown that the K_{ATP} channel is an important component of ischemic preconditioning (PC) in dogs (5,6). Therefore, based upon these results, there seems to be little doubt as to the potent cardioprotective effect that results from K_{ATP} channel activation during ischemia and that this channel plays an important endogenous protective function in the heart.

ISCHEMIC PRECONDITIONING

The phenomenon of ischemic preconditioning (PC) was first described by Murry *et al.* (8) in dogs. These authors found that four 5-minute periods of total coronary artery occlusion interspersed with 5-minute periods of reperfusion prior to a 40 minute occlusion period followed by 72 hours of reperfusion resulted in a marked (70-80%) reduction in myocardial infarct size when compared to a control group subjected to only 40 minutes of occlusion and 72 hours of reperfusion. Subsequently, Li *et al.* (9) demonstrated that one 5-minute period of occlusion produced a cardioprotective effect equivalent to that of six or twelve 5-minute preconditioning episodes in dogs. In almost all PC studies, single or multiple periods ranging from 3 to 10 minutes were sufficient to produce a PC-like effect (10). Furthermore, PC has consistently been shown to occur in all species in which it has been investigated including dogs, pigs, rabbits and rats and there is some recent evidence that it occurs in man (For reviews see ref 11).

Since the original discovery of ischemic PC, there has been intense interest in determining the mediators and subsequent cellular mechanisms involved in this remarkable cardioprotective phenomenon and some of these potential mediators, signal transduction pathways and end effectors are depicted in Figure 2.

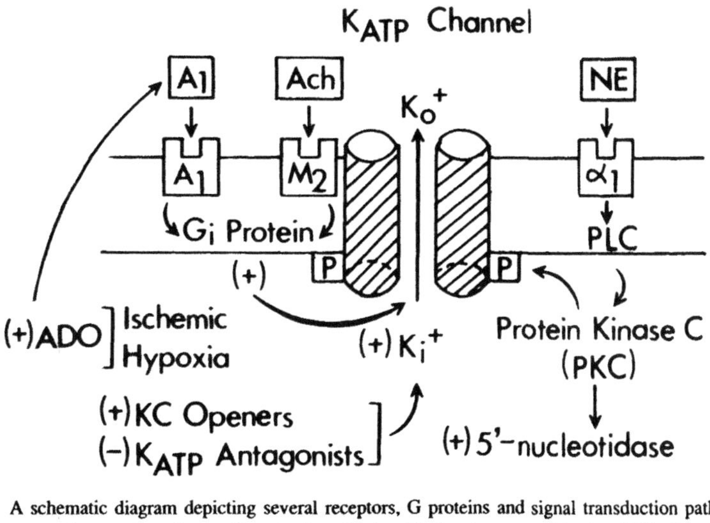

Figure 2. A schematic diagram depicting several receptors, G proteins and signal transduction pathways which have been proposed to mediate the cardioprotective effects of ischemic preconditioning (PC). Adenosine (ADO) and acetylcholine (Ach) have been shown to act via stimulation of the A1 or M2 receptor, respectively, which both activate a common G_i protein to turn on the ATP-sensitive K channel (K_{ATP}). Norepinephrine (NE) has been shown to mimic PC by combining with an $alpha_1$ (α_1) adrenergic receptor which activates the phospholipase C (PLC) - protein kinase C (PKC) cascade. Although speculative, some evidence suggests that PKC may phosphorylate the K_{ATP} channel and intensify or prolong its effects to protect the cardiac myocyte from ischemic damage.

Endogenous substances which have been shown to mimic ischemic PC include adenosine (12) and acetylcholine (13), known activators of G_i-protein-linked receptors and norepinephrine (4) which is known to activate the most commonly studied signal transduction mechanism which is the phospholipase C-protein kinase C pathway (14). Less is known concerning the possible end effectors responsible for PC but substantial support (5,6) has accumulated supporting a prominent role for the ATP-sensitive potassium channel (K_{ATP}) and the evidence for and against the role of the K_{ATP} channel in ischemic PC will be the major focus of this discussion.

When discussing potential mediators and/or effectors of ischemic PC, it is important to define a specific end point of injury which PC is protecting against since different mechanisms may be involved in the protection afforded by PC against infarction, stunning or cardiac arrhythmias (15). Murry *et al.* (8) initially defined ischemic PC as protection against myocardial necrosis, therefore infarct size will be the end point used in discussing the role of the K_{ATP} channel in this phenomenon. For those interested in the role of K_{ATP} channels in other models of PC with different end points, a recent review by Parratt and Kane (15) should be consulted.

THE ROLE OF THE K_{ATP} CHANNEL IN ISCHEMIC PRECONDITIONING

K_{ATP} Channels and PC in the Canine Heart:

The evidence supporting a role for the K_{ATP} channel in ischemic PC in the canine heart is substantial. In the initial studies from Gross' laboratory (50), they found that intravenous administration of glibenclamide, a specific K_{ATP} channel blocker, either before or immediately following a 5 minute period of ischemic PC, completely abolished its cardioprotective effect. The dose (0.3 mg/kg) of glibenclamide used had no effect on infarct size in nonpreconditioned dogs which suggests that this agent was selectively blocking the PC effect. It was also found that intravenous infusion of aprikalim, a selective K_{ATP} channel opener, at a nonhypotensive dose, markedly reduced infarct size to a degree nearly equivalent to that observed following ischemic PC, which further supported a role for K_{ATP} channels in this phenomenon. Subsequently, Auchampach *et al.* (6) infused the nonsulfonylurea K_{ATP} channel blocker, sodium 5-hydroxydecanoate (5-HD), intracoronary into nonpreconditioned or preconditioned dogs and found that this compound also antagonized the protective effect of PC without affecting infarct size in virgin hearts. In the same study, glibenclamide was administered intracoronary only during the 5 minute period of PC or only during the first 5 minutes of the prolonged 60 minute occlusion period and in both instances PC was totally abolished (Figure 3).

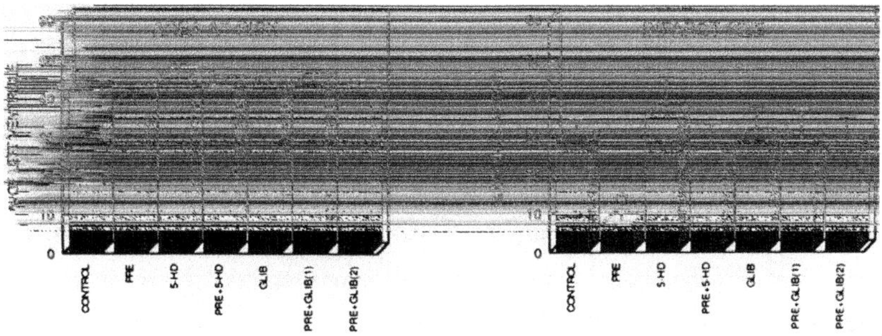

Figure 3. Graphs illustrating the effects of different treatments on the area at risk expressed as a percent of the left ventricle, and infarct size expressed as a percent of the area at risk in the canine heart. There were no differences between groups in area at risk, however, preconditioning (PRE) produced a significant reduction in infarct size (*$p<0.05$) as compared to the control nonpreconditioned group (CONTROL). Treatment with sodium- 5-hydroxydecanoate (PRE+5HD) during both the preconditioning occlusion and the first 5 minutes of the 60-minute occlusion period abolished the protective effect of preconditioning. Similarly, in preconditioned dogs, treatment with glibenclamide (GLIB), either during the 5-minute preconditioning occlusion [PRE+GLIB(1)] or the first 5 minutes of the 60-minute occlusion [PRE+GLIB(2)], abolished the protective effect of preconditioning on infarct size. Neither 5-HD nor glibenclamide had an effect on infarct size in the absence of preconditioning. Reprinted by permission from the British Medical Journal Publishing Group, from Auchampach *et al.* [6].

These results clearly indicated that opening of the K_{ATP} channel is not only necessary to trigger the PC response but also to maintain the protective effect over a finite period of time. Recent studies of Yao *et al.* (16) also support the idea that the K_{ATP} channel is a prime determinant of the memory phase of PC which normally last for 60-90 minutes following the PC stimulus in the canine heart. These authors (16) found that administration of glibenclamide 60 minutes following a 5-minute period of ischemic PC completely abolished the protective effect of PC which is normally observed at that time. Two other recent studies by Grover *et al.* (17) and Kitakaze *et al.* (18) also showed that intracoronary or intravenous administration of glibenclamide blocked the effect of ischemic PC in anesthetized dogs.

Studies in dogs using several K_{ATP} channel openers also indicate that these compounds can mimic the effect of ischemic PC to reduce infarct size. Mizumura *et al.* (19,20) have shown that nicorandil and bimakalim, 2 K_{ATP} channel openers, reduced infarct size in anesthetized dogs to a degree similar to that observed in our initial studies with aprikalim (5). In these later studies, nonhypotensive doses of bimakalim and nicorandil were administered intravenously prior to and during a 60 minute occlusion period. Using a different protocol, Gross and coworkers (unpublished results) and Kitakaze *et al.* (18) found that four 5-minute intracoronary infusions of 3 K_{ATP} channel openers, bimakalim, nicorandil or cromakalim, with intermittent 5 minute drug free periods, mimicked the effect of four 5-minute periods of ischemia separated by 5 minute periods of reperfusion to reduce infarct size in anesthetized dogs. In agreement, Yao and Gross (21) have demonstrated that adenosine and acetylcholine, acting via their A_1 and M_2 receptors could mimic the effects of ischemic PC and that these effects could be blocked by 5-HD (Figure 4). Finally, Mei and Gross (22) have recently shown that a brief period of regional hypoxia produces a reduction in infarct size similar to that of ischemic PC and that this effect could be blocked by glibenclamide. All of these findings strongly support a key role for K_{ATP} channels in ischemic PC in the canine heart.

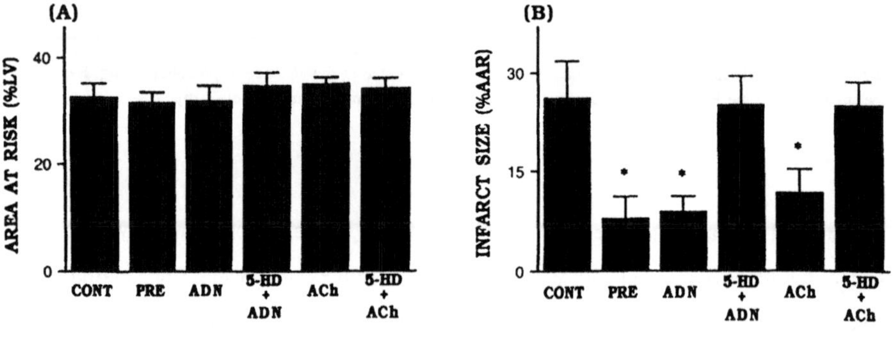

Figure 4. Graphs illustrating the effects of different treatments on the area at risk (AAR) expressed as a percent of the left ventricle (% LV) and infarct size expressed as a percent of the area at risk in the canine heart. There were no differences in area at risk between groups, however, preconditioning (PRE) produced by 10 minutes of ischemia or by a 10-minute intracoronary infusion of adenosine (400 µg/min, ADN) or acetylcholine (10 µg/min, ACh) produced a significant reduction in infarct size (*$p<0.05$) as compared to the control group (CONT). Concomitant treatment with the K_{ATP} channel antagonist, sodium 5-hydroxydecanoate (5-HD), with either adenosine or acetylcholine completely abolished their cardioprotective effects to reduce infarct size.

K_{ATP} CHANNELS AND PRECONDITIONING IN THE PORCINE HEART

Results obtained in the porcine heart support those obtained in dogs concerning an important role for the K_{ATP} channel in ischemic PC. Schultz *et al.* (23) recently reported that intravenous administration (0.5 mg/kg followed by 50 μg/min) of glibenclamide completely abolished the protective effect of PC. Glibenclamide had no effect on infarct size in non-preconditioned hearts. These authors also addressed potential mechanisms by which opening K_{ATP} channels might produce a cardioprotective effect and found that action potential shortening during the prolonged ischemic period in preconditioned hearts was accelerated as compared to the same time period in control hearts which suggests that the preconditioning stimulus sensitized the K_{ATP} channel to open more rapidly or to a greater extent during the prolonged ischemic interval. This is a necessary prerequisite if one is to make a strong case for the K_{ATP} channel in ischemic PC. In agreement, Rohmann *et al.* (24) have also shown that glibenclamide blocked ischemic PC in porcine hearts and that bimakalim, a selective K_{ATP} channel opener, markedly reduced infarct size (25). Thus, these results strongly support an important role for the K_{ATP} channel in ischemic PC in 2 large animal models, the dog and the pig. It should also be noted that the pig is a species with a sparse collateral circulation as compared to the dog and these results suggest that changes in collateral blood flow are not responsible or necessary for PC to occur.

K_{ATP} CHANNELS AND PRECONDITIONING IN RABBITS AND RATS

The results of studies concerning the role of K_{ATP} channels in ischemic PC in smaller animal species such as the rabbit and rat are not as unequivocal as those obtained in pigs and dogs. Thornton *et al.* (26) originally found in anesthetized rabbits that 3 doses of glibenclamide which produced large increases in infarct size in virgin hearts did not block the effects of ischemic PC. In contrast, Toombs *et al.* (27,28) found that glibenclamide completely blocked the effect of ischemic PC or the cardioprotective effects of adenosine in rabbits. The major difference in the studies of Thornton *et al.* [26] and Toombs *et al.* (27,28) was the anesthetic used, pentobarbital versus ketamine-xylazine, respectively. Since Haessler *et al.* (29) have recently shown that anesthetics per se can effect the intensity of the

PC response in rabbits, it is possible that this might explain the differences between the results of Thornton *et al.* (26) and Toombs *et al.* (27,28). However, since barbiturates have been used in all the dog studies and in the recent study of Kingma *et al.* (30) in rabbits where glibenclamide was shown to clearly block PC, it seems unlikely that the anesthetic is the sole reason for the differences observed between or within species.

Only one full-length paper has been published concerning the role of K_{ATP} channels in ischemic PC in rats. Liu and Downey (31) found that three 5-minute periods of ischemia produced PC in rat hearts and that this effect was not blocked by a dose (0.3 mg/kg) of glibenclamide that produced an increase in infarct size in nonpreconditioned hearts. In contrast, Qian *et al.* (32) recently reported that glibenclamide blocked both ischemic PC and the effect of acetylcholine to mimic PC in anesthetized rats although these findings were not supported by recent preliminary results of Richard *et al.* (33). Preliminary results from the laboratory of Gross (unpublished observations) showed that a novel K_{ATP} channel antagonist, U-37883, partially blocked the protective effect of three 5-minute periods of PC in anesthetized rats (see Figure 5). These differences in rats do not appear to be related to the anesthesia used. Obviously, further well-controlled studies are needed in the rat and rabbit to clarify the role of the K_{ATP} channel in ischemic PC in these 2 species.

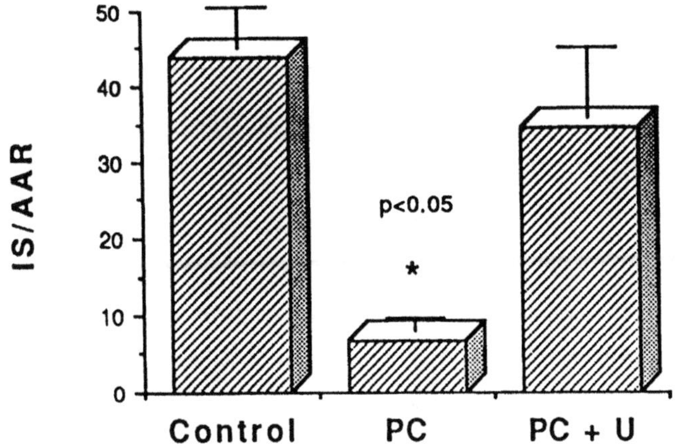

Figure 5. Graphs illustrating the effect of 3 five-minute periods of coronary artery occlusion interspersed with 5 minute periods of reperfusion prior to a prolonged 30 minute period of occlusion and 2 hours of reperfusion to precondition the intact rat heart. Preconditioning resulted in a reduction in infarct size (IS) expressed as a percent of the area at risk (AAR) from 44 ± 8 to 8 ± 3 %(*p<0.05). The specific K_{ATP} channel blocker, U37883 (U,6 mg/kg, iv) blocked the protective effects of ischemic PC (IS/AAR = 35 ± 8%).

K_{ATP} CHANNELS AND PRECONDITIONING IN MAN

Results suggestive of a role for the K_{ATP} channel in man have recently been obtained by Tomai *et al.* (34). These investigators clearly showed that one therapeutic dose (10 mg) of glibenclamide blocked a PC-like effect produced by consecutive 2 minute periods of coronary angioplasty separated by 5 minutes of reperfusion in patients with coronary artery disease. Obviously, since infarction was not the end point in these clinical studies, extrapolating these results to those obtained in infarct studies performed in animal models must be done with extreme caution, however, these results are certainly provocative.

In addition new data indicating a direct relationship between the K_{ATP} channel and preconditioning in human tissue has been obtained by Yellons' laboratory (see section below on the Role of Protein Kinase C)

MECHANISMS BY WHICH K_{ATP} CHANNELS MEDIATE PRECONDITIONING

Role of Enhanced Action Potential Shortening:

Only two studies have addressed the importance of the rate of action potential shortening during ischemia as a primary mechanism for the cardioprotective effect of K_{ATP} channel activation in ischemic PC (23,35). Tan *et al.* (35) found that action potential duration (APD) shortened to a greater extent during a prolonged ischemic period in isolated rabbit papillary muscle following a single 10 minute PC period. Similarly, Schultz *et al.* (23) demonstrated that APD shortening was accelerated during the first 10 minutes of a prolonged 90 minute ischemic period in porcine hearts which had been previously subjected to a single 10 minute period of ischemic PC. In support of these findings, preliminary results from Gross' laboratory in dogs also suggest that PC produced by 5 minutes of ischemia (Figure 6) results in an enhanced APD shortening during the initial 5 minutes of a prolonged 60 minute ischemic period. APD shortening and the infarct-limiting effect of ischemic PC were both blocked by the K_{ATP} antagonist, glibenclamide.

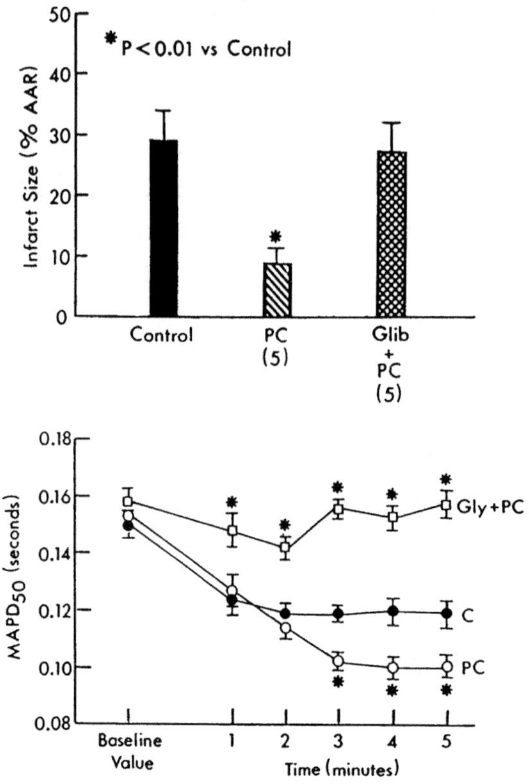

Figure 6. Graphs illustrating the effect of 5 minutes of ischemic preconditioning (PC) on infarct size expressed as a percent of the area at risk (AAR) in dog hearts subjected to 60 minutes of coronary artery occlusion and 4 hours of reperfusion (upper graph) and the effect of PC on the rate of monophasic action potential shortening (lower graph) expressed as the monophasic action potential duration (seconds) at 50% repolarization ($MAPD_{50}$). PC resulted in a marked reduction in infarct size and enhanced the rate of $MAPD_{50}$ shortening during the initial 5 minutes of the prolonged 60 minute ischemic period (*$p<0.05$). The K_{ATP} channel antagonist, glibenclamide (Glib, Gly) completely blocked the beneficial effect of ischemic PC.

On the other hand, Gross has previously demonstrated that a dissociation exists between the rate of APD shortening and the cardioprotective effect of the selective K_{ATP} opener bimakalim (36). These data suggest that enhanced APD shortening is not essential for the cardioprotective effect of K_{ATP} activation during ischemia, however, since the mechanism of action of PC and K_{ATP} openers may not be identical, it is difficult to assess the importance of APD shortening in these 2 situations. Obviously, further studies are necessary in which APD shortening is prevented by pharmacological agents which prolong APD to determine the essential role of APD shortening in the PC response.

THE ROLE OF MITOCHONDRIAL K_{ATP} CHANNELS

Several studies (37,38) have recently demonstrated the presence of an ATP-dependent K^+ channel in the inner mitochondrial membrane in rat liver and bovine hearts (see Figure 1). These channels were shown to be reversibly inactivated by ATP applied to the matrix side during an inside-out patch configuration and were shown to be inhibited by glibenclamide. More recently, Paucek *et al.* (39) demonstrated that the mitochondrial K_{ATP} channel could be activated by GTP or GTP-γS as well as by several K_{ATP} channel openers such as diazoxide and cromakalim. Although the function of this channel under normal and ischemic conditions is presently unknown, it is intriguing to speculate that this channel, in addition to the sarcolemmal K_{ATP} channel, may play an important role in the potent anti-ischemic actions of K_{ATP} openers and PC and may help explain the dissociation which we have previously observed between the infarct size limiting effect of bimakalim and the rate of APD shortening (36). The recent development of several novel cardioselective K_{ATP} openers which are cardioprotective in the absence of enhanced APD shortening support this possibility (40). Also see chapter by Grover. Whether the mitochondrial K_{ATP} channel plays a role in ischemic or hypoxic PC awaits further studies.

THE ROLE OF PROTEIN KINASE C (PKC)

Recent evidence obtained in rat and rabbit hearts clearly suggest an important role for PKC in initiating as well as maintaining the protective effect of ischemic PC (41,42,43). Subsequent to PKC activation, it has been proposed that an intracellular protein that this enzyme might phosphorylate and activate is the K_{ATP} channel (see Figure 2). Phosphorylation of this channel could ultimately be responsible for the memory phase of PC which has recently been attributed to the K_{ATP} channel (16). In support of this hypothesis, DeWeille *et al.* (3) have demonstrated that stimulation of PKC in rat insulinoma cells by somatostatin or a phorbol ester, phorbol myristate acetate (PMA), results in activation of the K_{ATP} channel. In addition, Yellons' group have shown (44,45) that it is possible to both precondition and protect human atrial muscle with hypoxia and cromakalim respectively (45)

as well as directly with the PKC agonist 1,2-dioctonoyl-sn-glycerol (DG) (44,46) in human and rabbit heart respectivelly. In addition, this preconditioning effect can be abolished with the specific PKC inhibitor, chelerythrine (44). Furthermore exciting studies using this human muscle preparation quite clearly show that this preconditioning effect with the PKC agonist (DG) is blocked by the K_{ATP} channel blocker glibenclamide (47). *These results clearly demonstrate for the first time that the effector protein in the human muscle, appears to be the K_{ATP} channel.* Interestingly, similar studies in the rabbit using the same PKC agonists and antagonists as well as the K_{ATP} channel opener cromakalim, and blocker, glibenclamide, were unable to demonstrate that the end effector for protection was the K_{ATP} channel (46). Thus it appears, as indicated earlier, that the rabbit, although able to be preconditioned with ischemia and "protected" with K_{ATP} channel openers, K_{ATP} channel opening itself is not essential for preconditioning in this species.
Interestingly, Harding *et al.* (48) have also shown that polymixin B, a compound which has been shown to block ischemic PC in rabbit hearts (42), blocks the K_{ATP} channel as well as PKC in insulin-secreting cells.

Although PKC activation has not been shown to be associated with ischemic PC in dogs or pigs, more studies are clearly needed in these species to confirm or rule out an interaction between the K_{ATP} channel and PKC. However, as mentioned above, it is encouraging to see that such an interaction appears to occur in the human muscle.

THE ROLE OF G PROTEINS AND MEMBRANE RECEPTORS IN PRECONDITIONING

Another possible mechanism by which the K_{ATP} channel may be sensitized to the effect produced by a short ischemic stimulus sufficient to PC the heart may be via the activation of specific membrane receptors and G proteins.

The first study to suggest that K_{ATP} channels are linked to the A_1 adenosine receptor by a G_i protein was performed by Kirsch *et al.* (49) in excised membrane patches obtained from neonatal rat ventricular myocytes. These authors found that application of 0.1 mM ATP to the intracellular side of membrane patches inhibited K_{ATP} channel activity whereas addition of 0.1 mM of GTP-γS restored K_{ATP} activity. Addition of 0.1 mM GTP plus either 10 μM of extracellular adenosine or 100 nM of the selective A_1 receptor agonist, cyclohexyladenosine, activated the channel similar to that observed with GTP-γS. It was also found that several subunits of G_α mimicked the effect of GTP-γS. In contrast, $alpha_o$ or G_s did not mimic the effect of GTP-gammaS which suggested that the adenosine A_1 receptor is linked to the K_{ATP} channel via a $G_i\alpha$ pathway. In agreement, Ito *et al.* (50) and Kurachi *et al.* (51) found that GTP in the presence of adenosine and GTP-γS produced an increase in K_{ATP} channel activity in inside-out patches obtained from guinea pig ventricular myocytes. Furthermore, Ito *et al.* (52) demonstrated that $G_i\alpha$'s activated the K_{ATP} channel which was phosphorylated by 100 μM Mg • ATP. Gßγ inhibited the effect of adenosine to activate the K_{ATP} channel in the presence of intracellular GTP. More recently, Ito *et al.* (52) suggested that G_i proteins stimulate myocardial K_{ATP} channels by decreasing the inhibitory potency of ATP and that adenosine and acetylcholine mimic or enhance this effect. All of these results suggest that adenosine or ischemic preconditioning may produce their cardioprotective effects via an adenosine A_1 receptor-mediated G_i protein-linked activation of the K_{ATP} channel. That acetylcholine also has been shown to mimic the effects of ischemic PC and is known to act via a similar G_i protein in ventricular cells as adenosine supports this hypothesis. Further support for a role of the G_i protein in ischemic PC has been furnished by Thornton et al (53) and Ichihara *et al.* (54) who showed that pertussis toxin abolished the effect of PC in rabbit and canine hearts. These results obtained in isolated membrane patches *in vitro* and in whole animals are strongly suggestive of an important link between G_i protein-linked membrane receptors such as the adenosine A_1 receptor and the K_{ATP} channel in mediating the cardioprotective effects of exogenous adenosine and its analogues as well as ischemic PC.

Several studies performed in vivo also suggest that there is an important link between adenosine A1 receptors and the K_{ATP} channel in mediating PC (17,55). Initially Grover et al (17) found that intracoronary administration of the selective A1 receptor agonist R-PIA, reduced infarct size in dogs and that this protective effect was abolished by glibenclamide.

Although indirect, these results were the first to suggest a link between adenosine A_1 receptors and the K_{ATP} channel in ischemic PC in vivo. Concurrently, Auchampach and Gross (55) showed that a 5 minute intracoronary infusion of exogenous adenosine plus dipyridamole, an adenosine uptake blocker, significantly reduced myocardial infarct size and that this effect was blocked by glibenclamide. These results also suggested that activation of adenosine A1 receptors produces myocardial PC by opening K_{ATP} channels. In a more recent study in dogs, Yao and Gross (21) showed that a 10 minute intracoronary infusion of adenosine produced a reduction in myocardial infarct size similar to that of 10 minutes of ischemic PC. When glibenclamide was administered 15 minutes prior to the adenosine infusion or another selective K_{ATP} channel antagonist, 5-hydroxydecanoate (5-HD) was infused concomitantly with adenosine into the left anterior descending coronary artery for 10 minutes, the PC-like effect of adenosine was abolished. These data further support the idea that adenosine mediates its cardioprotective effect via a cardiac K_{ATP} channel-linked mechanism.

More recently, Toombs et al. (27, 28) showed that glibenclamide reversed the protective effects of ischemic PC in anesthetized rabbits and that a low dose of glibenclamide completely blocked the cardioprotective effect of exogenously administered adenosine. A higher dose of glibenclamide also blocked the protection afforded by adenosine treatment, however, infarct size in non-preconditioned hearts was increased by this dose. These authors concluded that part of the cardioprotective effect of adenosine in rabbit hearts was the result of K_{ATP} channel activation.

Finally, in a recent study in anesthetized swine, Van Winkle and co-workers (52) further tested the hypothesis that adenosine A_1 receptor-mediated cardioprotection is the result of K_{ATP} channel activation. These authors demonstrated that intracoronary infusion of adenosine and of R-PIA, an adenosine A1 receptor agonist, produced marked reductions in myocardial infarct size. In the case of R-PIA, the cardioprotective effect was completely blocked by sodium 5-hydroxydecanoate (5-HD). These authors concluded that both adenosine A_1 receptors and K_{ATP} channels may be involved in ischaemic PC in pigs.

SUMMARY

In summary, we believe that the vast majority of studies performed in intact animals in which myocardial infarct size is used as the end point to define the cardioprotective effect of ischemic PC *support a key role for the K_{ATP} channel as both a trigger and as an end effector in this phenomenon.* Future studies are necessary in isolated myocyte models of PC and by use of whole cell and single channel patch clamp technology to further understand the mechanisms, i.e., receptors, signal transduction pathways, ion channels, enzymes, involved in producing the potent cardioprotective effect resulting from K_{ATP} channel activation. In this regard, preliminary results of Liu *et al.* (57) have shown that the K_{ATP} opener, pinacidil, mimics the effects of ischemic PC in an isolated rabbit myocyte model, however, this protective effect of pinacidil was blocked by 8-SPT, a nonselective adenosine receptor antagonist. These results are provocative and further support the hypothesis that K_{ATP} channels and adenosine interact by some unknown mechanism to elicit ischemic PC.
In addition the results from Yellons' group (45,47) indicating a direct role for the K_{ATP} channel as the end effector in preconditioning in human muscle are encouraging to say the least. Finally, a recent study by Ashford *et al.* (58) in which the K_{ATP} channel has been cloned in rat myocardium suggest that new molecular approaches will soon be available to help us better understand the factors modulating K_{ATP} channel activity under normal and ischemic conditions.

ACKNOWLEDGEMENTS

The authors wish to thank Anna Hsu, Jeannine Moore and Carol Knapp for their excellent technical assistance, artwork and typing in the preparation of this chapter. The research results reported from Gross' laboratory were supported by USPHS grant HL 08311. and that from Yellons' laboratory were supported by the British Heart Foundation, the Wellcome Trust and the Hatter Foundation.

REFERENCES

1. Noma A. 1983. ATP-regulated K^+ channels in cardiac muscle. Nature 305: 147-148.

2. Nichols CG, Lederer WJ. 1991. Adenosine-triphosphate sensitive potassium channels in the cardiovascular system. Am J Physiol 262: H1675-H1686.

3. DeWeille JR, Schmid-Antomarchi H, Fosset M, Lazdunski M. 1989. Regulation of ATP-sensitive K^+ channels in insulinoma cells. Activation by somatostatin and protein kinase C and the role of cAMP. Proc Natl Acad Sci USA 86: 2971-2975.

4. Cole WG, McPherson CD, Sontag D. 1991. ATP-regulated K^+ channels protect the myocardium against ischemia/reperfusion damage. Circ Res 69: 571-581.

5. Gross GJ, Auchampach JA. 1992. Blockade of ATP-sensitive potassium channels prevents myocardial preconditioning in dogs. Circ Res 70: 223-233.

6. Auchampach JA, Grover GJ, Gross GJ. 1992. Blockade of ischemic preconditioning in dogs by the novel ATP dependent potassium channel antagonist 5-hydroxydecanoate. Cardiovasc Res 26: 1054-1062.

7. Auchampach JA, Maruyama M, Cavero I, Gross GJ. 1992. Pharmacological evidence for a role of ATP-regulated potassium channels in myocardial stunning. Circulation 86: 311-319.

8. Murry CE, Jennings RB, Reimer KA. 1986. Preconditioning with ischemia: a delay of lethal cell injury in ischemic myocardium. Circulation 74: 1124-1136.

9. Li GC, Vasquesz JA, Gallagher KP, Lucchesi BR. 1990. Myocardial protection with preconditioning. Circulation 82: 609-619.

10. Walker DM, Yellon DM. 1992. Ischemic preconditioning: from mechanisms to exploitation. Cardiovasc Res 26: 734-739.

11. Kloner RA, Yellon DM. 1994.Does ischemic preconditioning occur in patients? J Am Coll Cardiol 1994; 24: 1133-1142.

12. Liu GS, Thornton JD, Van Winkle DM, Stanley AWH, Olsson RA, Downey JM. 1991. Protection against infarction afforded by preconditioning is mediated via A_1 adenosine receptors in rabbit heart. Circulation 84: 350-356.

13. Yao Z, Gross GJ. 1993. Acetylcholine mimics ischemic preconditioning via a glibenclamide-sensitive mechanism in dogs. Am J Physiol 264: H2221-H2225.

14. Tsuchida A, Liu Y, Liu GS, Cohen MV, Downey JM. 1994. a_1-adrenergic agonists precondition rabbit ischemic myocardium independent of adenosine by direct activation of protein kinase C. Circ Res 75: 576-585.

15. Parratt JR, Kane KA. 1994. K_{ATP} channels in ischaemic preconditioning Cardiovasc Res 28: 783-787.

16. Yao Z, Mizumura T, Mei D, Gross GJ. 1994. Activation of K_{ATP} channels may play a role in the "memory" of ischemic preconditioning (PC) in anesthetized dogs. Circulation 90: 573.

17. Grover GJ, Sleph PG, Dzwonczyk S. 1992. Role of myocardial ATP-sensitive potassium channels in mediating preconditioning in the dog heart and their possible interaction with adenosine A_1 receptors. Circulation 86: 1310-1316.

18. Kitakaze M, Komamura K, Chujo M, Mori H, Hori M. 1994. Role of ectosolic 5^1 nucleotidase activation in the infarct size-limiting effect mediated by the opening of K^+ channels: implications for ischemic preconditioning. Circulation 90: 574.

19. Mizumura T, Nithipatikom K, Gross GJ. 1995. Effects of nicorandil and glycerlyl trinitrate on infarct size, adenosine release and neutrophil infiltration in the dog. Cardiovasc Res 29: 482-489.

20. Mizumura T, Nithipatikom K, Gross GJ. 1995. Bimakalim, an ATP-sensitive potassium channel opener, mimics the effects of ischemic preconditioning to reduce infarct size, adenosine release and neutrophil function in dogs. Circulation (In Press).

21. Yao Z, Gross GJ. 1994. A comparison of adenosine-induced cardioprotection and ischemic preconditioning in dogs: Efficacy, time course and role of K_{ATP} channels. Circulation 89: 1229-1236.

22. Mei D, Gross GJ. 1995. Evidence for the involvement of the ATP-sensitive potassium channel in a novel model of hypoxic preconditioning in dogs. Cardiovasc Res (In Press).

23. Schultz R, Rose J, Heusch G. 1994. Involvement of activation of ATP-dependent potassium channels is involved in ischemic preconditioning in swine. Am J Physiol 267: H1341-H1352.

24. Rohmann S, Weygandt H, Schelling P, Soei LK, Verdouw PD, Lues I. 1994. Involvement of ATP-sensitive potassium channels in preconditioning protection. Basic Res Cardiol 89: 563-576.

25. Rohmann S, Weygandt H, Schelling P, Soei LK, Becker KH, Verdouw PD, Lues I, Hausler G. 1994. Effect of bimakalim (EMD 52692) an opener of ATP sensitive potassium channels on infarct size, coronary blood flow, regional wall function, and oxygen consumption in swine. Cardiovasc Res 28: 858-863.

26. Thornton JD, Thornton CS, Sterling DL, Downey JM. 1993. Blockade of ATP-sensitive potassium channels increases infarct size but does not prevent preconditioning in rabbit hearts. Circ Res 72: 44-49.

27. Toombs CF, Moore TL, Shebuski RJ. 1993. Limitation of infarct size in the rabbit by ischemic preconditioning is reversible with glibenclamide. Cardiovasc Res 27: 617-622.

28. Toombs CF, McGee DS, Johnston WE, Vinten-Johansen J. 1993. Protection from ischaemic-reperfusion injury with adenosine pretreatment is reversed by inhibition of ATP-sensitive potassium channels. Cardiovasc Res 27: 623-629.

29. Haessler R, Kuzume K, Chien GL, Wolff RA, Davis RF, VanWinkle DM. 1994. Anaesthetics alter the magnitude of infarct limitation by ischaemic preconditioning. Cardiovasc Res 28: 1574-1580.

30. Kingma JG Jr, Hazenberg M, Simard D, Rouleau JR. 1994. Interactions between adenosine and ATP-sensitive potassium channels during ischemic preconditioning. J Mol Cell Cardiol 26: no 6.(abst) CL1

31. Liu Y, Downey JM. 1992. Ischemic preconditioning protects against infarction in rat hearts. Am J Physiol 263: H1107-H1112.

32. Q¢uian YZ, Levasseur J, Yoshida JK, Jesse RL, Hess ML, Kukreja RC. 1994. Acetylcholine partially preconditions rat hearts by a glibenclamide-sensitive mechanism. FASEB J 8: 747.

33. Richard V, Blanc T, Tron C, Thuillez C. 1994. Acetylcholine limits infarct size through muscarinic receptor stimulation and production of nitric oxide but does not contribute to preconditioning in rats.

34. Tomai F, Crea F, Caspardone A, Versaci F, DePaulis R, Penta de Peppo A, Chiariello L, Gioffre¢. 1994. Ischemic preconditioning during coronary angioplasty is prevented by glibenclamide, a selective ATP-sensitive K^+ channel blocker. Circulation 90: 700-705.

35. Tan HL, Mazon P, Verberne HJ, Sleeswijk ME, Coronel R, Opthof T, Janse MJ. 1993. Ischaemic preconditioning delays ischaemia-induced uncoupling in rabbit myocardium by activation of ATP-sensitive potassium channels. Cardiovasc Res 27: 644-651.

36. Yao Z, Gross GJ. 1994. Effects of the K_{ATP} channel opener bimakalim on coronary blood flow, monophasic action potential duration and infarct size in dogs. Circulation 89: 1769-1775.

37. Inoue I, Nagase H, Kishi K, Higuti T. 1991. ATP-sensitive K^+ channel in the mitochondrial inner membrane. Nature 352: 244-247.

38. Paucek P, Mironova G, Mahdi F, Beavis AD, Woldegiorgis G, Garlid K. 1992. Reconstitution and partial purification of the glibenclamide-sensitive, ATP-dependent K^+ channel from rat liver and beef heart mitochondria. J Biol Chem 267: 26062-26069.

39. Paucek P, Yarov-Yorovoy V, Sun X, Garlid KD. 1995. Physiological and pharmacological activators of the mitochondrial K_{ATP} channel. Biophysics J 60: A145.

40. Atwal KS, Grover GJ, Ahmed SZ, Ferrara FN, Harper TW, Kim KS, Sleph PG, Dzwonczyk S, Russell AD, Moreland S, McCullough JR, Normandin DE. 1993. Cardioselective anti-ischemic ATP-sensitive potassium channel openers. J Med Chem 36: 3971-3974.

41. Speechly-Dick ME, Mocanu MM, Yellon DM. 1994. Protein Kinase C - Its role in ischaemic preconditioning in the rat. Circ Res 1994 75: 586-590.

42. Liu Y, Ytrehus K, Downey JM. 1994. Evidence that translocation of protein kinase C is a key event during ischemic preconditioning of rabbit myocardium. J Mol Cell Cardiol 26: 661-668.

43. Ytrehus K, Liu Y, Downey JM. 1994. Preconditioning protects ischemic rabbit heart by protein kinase C activation. Am J Physiol 266: H1145-H1152.

44 Speechly-Dick ME, Yellon DM. 1995. Ichaemic preconditioning in human myocardium: the role of protein kinase C. Brit Heart J 1995 (abst)

45 Speechly-Dick ME, Grover GJ, Yellon DM. 1995. The ATP-sensitive potassium channel: its role in ischaemic preconditioning in human atrial trabecula. J Mol Cell Cardiol (In Press) abst.

46 Jenkins DP, Kerac M, Yellon DM. 1995. Preconditioning: Protein Kinase C and the K_{ATP} channel in the isolated rabbit heart. J Mol Cell Cardiol (In Press) abst.

47 Speechly-Dick ME, Grover G, Yellon DM. 1995. Does Ischemic preconditioning in the human atrium involve Protein kinase C and the ATP-dependent K channel? Studies of contractile function in an in vitro model.
Circ Res (In Press)

48. Harding EA, Jaggar JH, Squires PE, Dunne MJ. 1993. Protein kinase C and the modulation of ATP-sensitive potassium channels in insulin-secreting cells. Biochem Soc Trans 21: 3885.

49. Kirsch GE, Codina J, Birnbaumer L, Brown AM. 1990. Coupling of ATP-sensitive K^+ channels to A_1 receptors by G proteins in rat ventricular myocytes. Am J Physiol 259: H820-H826.

50. Ito H, Tung RT, Sugimoto T, Kobayashi I, Takahashi K, Katada T, Vi M, Kurachi Y. 1992. On the mechanism of G protein ßg subunit activation of the muscarinic K^+ channel in guinea pig atrial cell membrane. Comparison with the ATP-sensitive K+ channel. J Gen Physiol 99: 961-983.

51. Kurachi Y, Tung RT, Ito H, Nakajima T. 1992. G protein activation of cardiac muscarinic K^+ channels. Prog Neurobiol 39: 229-246.

52. Ito H, Verecke J, Carmeliet E. 1994. Mode of regulation by G protein of the ATP-sensitive K^+ channel in guinea pig ventricular cell membrane. J Physiol 478.1: 101-108.

53. Thornton JD, Liu GS, Downey JM. 1993. Pretreatment with pertussis toxin blocks the protective effects of preconditioning: evidence for Gi-protein mechanism. J Mol Cell Cardiol 25: 311-320.

54. Ichihara K, Miura K, Nakai T, Satoh K. 1994. Effect of preconditioning on myocardial pH during ischemia in dogs. J Mol Cell Cardiol 26: 66.

55. Auchampach JA, Gross GT. 1993. Adenosine A1 receptors, K_{ATP} channels and ischemic preconditioning in dogs. Am J Physiol 224: H1327-H1336.

56. Van Winkle DM, Chien GL, Wolfe RA, Soifer BE, Kuzume K, Davis RF. 1994. Cardioprotection provided by adenosine receptor activation is abolished by the blockade of the K_{ATP} channel. Am J Physiol 166: H829-H839.

57. Liu GS, Ganote CE, Downey JM. 1994. Activation of adenosine receptors is required for protection from a direct opener of K_{ATP} channels in rabbit ventricular myocytes. Circulation 90: 2570.

58. Ashford MLJ, Bond CT, Blair TA, Adelman JP. 1994. Cloning and functional expression of a rat heart K_{ATP} channel. Nature 370: 456-459.

5

POTASSIUM CHANNEL ACTIVATION AND ARRHYTHMOGENICITY

MICHIEL J JANSE and ARTHUR A M WILDE.
Department of Experimental & Clinical Cardiology, M-0-52, Academic Medical Center, University of Amsterdam, P.O.Box 22700, 1100 De Amsterdam, The Netheralands.

INTRODUCTION

It may be expected that potassium channel openers (KCOs), in particular openers of the ATP sensitive K^+ channel, will become increasingly available for the treatment of angina pectoris and hypertension. It is therefore important to define possible proarrhythmic effects of KCOs especially in the setting of acute ischemia. As will be shown there are surprisingly few experimental data allowing a firm conclusion be made regarding this important issue. A discussion about pro- and anti-arrhythmic effects of KCOs is confounded by a number of factors, of which the most important are: dosage, species differences, experimental models (notably in vivo experiments versus experiments on isolated preparations or myocytes), heart rate, and in the setting of ischaemia the time after coronary artery occlusion. We will firstly discuss the effects of KCOs on normoxic cardiac tissue before focusing on ischaemia-induced arrhythmias.

EFFECTS OF K-CHANNEL ACTIVATION ON NORMOXIC CARDIAC TISSUE

The most prominent electrophysiological effect of activation of K-channels is a shortening of the action potential duration, and thus a shortening of the refractory period. Shortening of the refractory period will shorten the wavelength (i.e. the product of conduction velocity and refractory period), which promotes the occurrence of re-entrant arrhythmias (1)
In open-chest dogs, KCOs cause only a significant shortening of both atrial and ventricular refractory periods at doses that reduce mean arterial blood pressure by 30 to 40% or more (2,3). When these changes occurred, either by application of strongly hypotensive doses or by intracoronary injection of high doses, atrial (2,3) and ventricular arrhythmias (3,4,5) did indeed occur. In addition in isolated guinea pig hearts, very high concentrations of pinacidil were required to demonstrate an increased propensity for spontaneous and electrically induced arrhythmias (6).

Maximal plasma concentrations of nicorandil in humaans after oral administration are between 2 and 8 uM, those of pinacidil lower than 1 uM (7,8). Such concentrations do not activate K_{ATP} channels in isolated myocytes (9, 10), nor do they shorten the action potential in isolated guinea pig myocytes (11) or isolated canine Purkinje fiber preparations (12). However, similar doses (1-5 uM pinacidil) did induce electrophysiological inhomogeneities in isolated endo- and epicardial canine preparations (13). In endocardial cells, only a small reduction in action potential duration was observed. In contrast, epicardial cells responded in a nonhomogeneous fashion: either action potential duration was markedly shortened, with loss of their characteristic spike-and-dome configuration, or only a minor shortening was induced. These changes occurred specifically at very slow rates of stimulation (cycle lengths in the order of 2,000 msec). Premature stimulation caused re-entrant extrasystoles, and spontaneous re-entry was also observed. These arrhythmias could be abolished by addition of glibenclamide (a blocker of the ATP-sensitive K-channel) or by 4-aminopyridine (a blocker of the transient outward current) (13). It remains to be seen whether such marked inhomogeneities can be induced by similar doses in the in vivo heart at physiological heart rates.

Therapeutic doses do affect repolarisation in humans, because ST-segment changes in the electrocardiogram have been observed after treatment with pinacidil (14,15).

However, since clinical trials with KCOs, tested as anti-anginal or anti-hypertensive agents, did not report proarrhythmic effects (8,16), it may be concluded that in therapeutic doses KCOs are unlikely to cause arrhythmias in nonischemic hearts. *In fact, it could be postulated that in nonhypotensive doses KCOs may be anti-arrhythmic.* In normal Purkinje fibers, with high levels of maximal diastolic potential, KCOs suppress spontaneous diastolic depolarisation (12,17,18,19) and reduce the rate of idioventricular rhythm in the intact ventricle (20). Thus, KCOs would be effective against arrhythmias caused by enhanced normal automaticity in the Purkinje system, such as ventricular extrasystoles and some idiopathic ventricular tachycardias (21,22)

Abnormal automaticity is spontaneous impulse formation occurring in partially depolarised cells that normally have a resting membrane potential between -80 and -90 mV. Ectopic atrial tachycardias and accelerated idioventricular rhythms in the subacute phase of myocardial infarction are caused by abnormal automaticity (21,22). Because KCOs hyperpolarise the membrane, they abolish abnormal automaticity (12,17,19). In dogs with an experimental infarction, the arrhythmias occurring during the subacute phase (i.e. several hours to 3 days following coronary artery occlusion), which are caused by abnormal automaticity in surviving Purkinje fibers were decreased by KCOs (23).

Delayed afterdepolarisations should be diminished by activation of K- channels because the hyperpolarising K current will counteract the inward current responsible for the delayed afterdepolarisation. Experiments in in vitro preparations did indeed show that delayed afterdepolarisations, induced by high extracellular calcium concentrations or cardiac glycosides, were either diminished or abolished (17,18,19). In contrast, KCOs were not effective in abolishing triggered arrhythmias based on delayed afterdepolarisations in in vivo experiments (24,25). Clinical arrhythmias caused by delayed-afterdepolarisations-induced triggered activity include the arrhythmias associated with digitalis intoxication and catecholamine-dependent ventricular tachycardia (21,22)

Arrhythmias caused by early afterdepolarisations occur in situations where action potential duration is prolonged, such as bradycardia, hypokalemia, exposure to drugs that prolong the action potential (K-channel blockers), the long QT syndrome. Torsade de pointes, which occurs in these situations, is thought to be due to, or at least initiated by, triggered activity based on early afterdepolarisations (21,22). K-channel activation will accelerate repolarisation and may be expected to abolish early afterdepolarisations. Both in vivo and in vitro experiments showed that the occurrence of early afterdepolarisations and Torsade de pointes was reduced or prevented by KCOs (26-30). Surprisingly, the anti-arrhythmic effect could be obtained at doses which did not shorten the prolonged action potential (26,29) although in dogs treated with d-Sotalol the anti-arrhythmic effect was indeed accompanied by a normalisation of the QT-interval (28).

In summary, activation of K-channels is effective against arrhythmias that are caused by disturbances in impulse formation, i.e. enhanced normal and abnormal automaticity and triggered activity due to early and delayed afterdepolarisations. *On a theoretical basis one could predict that K-channel activation could be both pro- and anti-arrhythmic for re-entrant arrhythmias.* A short wavelength, which predisposes to re-entry, can be the result of a shortening of the refractory period (or action potential duration), slowing of conduction, or both. K-channel activation resulting in a marked shortening of the action potential could be pro-arrhythmic. If, on the other hand, a re-entrant circuit has a segment of partially depolarised tissue resulting in slow conduction, the hyperpolarising effect of K-channel activation could increase conduction velocity, and thus prolong the wavelength, which would be an anti-arrhythmic action. As discussed above, the available experimental evidence indicates that in normoxic hearts in vivo, only high doses of KCOs, which are hypotensive, cause shortening of the action potential and induce arrhythmias that are presumably re-entrant. To our knowledge, there is no experimental evidence that supports an eventual anti-re-entrant action.

EFFECTS OF K-CHANNEL ACTIVATION ON ISCHAEMIC MYOCARDIUM

Before discussing whether or not KCOs are proarrhythmic in the setting of acute ischaemia, it is important to describe some characteristics of ischaemia-induced ventricular arrhythmias.

In hearts of large experimental animals, such as dogs and pigs, ventricular arrhythmias during the first hour of regional ischaemia occur in two distinct periods (for references see 31 and 32). After the onset of ischaemia an early phase (IA) lasts from about 2 to 10 minutes. Following an arrhythmia free period, a second phase (IB) starts at about 15 to 20 minutes and lasts until 30 to 50 minutes. After the first hour, arrhythmias subside until the delayed arrhythmias of the subacute phase appear after several to 24 hours (31, 32). This phase may last for several days. In smaller species, such as rats, guinea pigs, cats and rabbits, a unimodal rather than a bimodal distribution is usually observed during the first 30 minutes of both regional and global ischaemia (33,34,35,36) where the arrhythmias start after 6 minutes, peak between 10 to 12 minutes and sub-side after 15 minutes. Most likely, these arrhythmias correspond to the phase IB arrhythmias of larger animals. It is important to make a distinction between these three phases of arrhythmias (IA, IB and the delayed phase of subacute infarction) because the arrhythmia mechanisms are not the same, nor are the electrophysiological changes that form the basis of the arrhythmias. As already mentioned, abnormal automaticity in partially depolarised Purkinje fibres overlying the developing infarct is the dominant arrhythmia mechanism of the delayed phase (31,32) and KCOs are effective in suppressing these arrhythmias (23). The mechanisms for the IB arrhythmias are unknown. Their occurrence coincides with the time that ischaemic cells become electrically uncoupled. The slow and inhomogeneous conduction that is the consequence of an increased coupling resistance may be a factor causing re-entry. The dominant mechanism for ventricular tachycardia and fibrillation during the IA phase is re-entry.

The most important electrophysiological alterations that set the stage for re-entry in the IA phase are slowing of conduction velocity and inhomogeneities in excitability, largely caused by inhomogeneities in extracellular K^+ concentration (31,37). Although action potential duration of ischaemic cells shortens, this does not automatically mean that refractory periods shorten as well. In partially depolarised ischaemic cells, recovery of excitability lags behind completion of repolarisation. Because of this so-called post-repolarisation-refractoriness, refractory periods in the centre of the ischaemic zone (where extracellular K^+ concentrations are highest and resting membrane potential is greatly reduced) are actually longer than in normal myocardium. Closer to the border with normal tissue, where extracellular K^+ concentrations are lower and resting membrane potential is less depressed, refractory periods may be shorter than those of non-ischaemic myocardium. As a general rule, re-entry is facilitated by a shortening of the wavelength, the product of conduction velocity and refractory period. The concern that KCOs might be pro-arrhythmic during the hyperacute phase of ischaemia is based on the concept that they produce a further shortening of the action potential of ischaemic cells, and a shortening of the refractory period, and thereby a shortening of the wavelength.

On purely theoretical grounds, it is by no means certain that KCOs, even when they shorten the action potential of ischaemic cells, also shorten their refractory period. When, for instance, KCOs would enhance K^+ efflux, and extracellular K concentration would increase, resting membrane potential would be more depolarised and post-repolarisation-refractoriness would be prolonged.

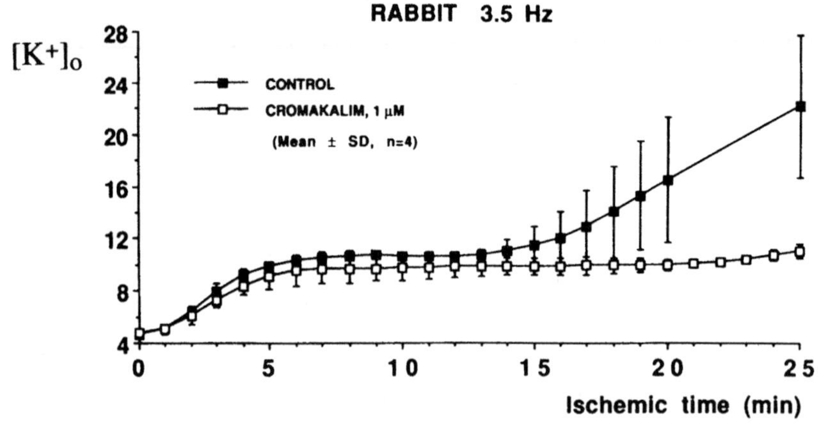

Figure 1. Extracellular potassium concentration ($[K^+]_0$) in the absence (closed symbols, n=4) and presence of 1 mM cromakalim (open symbols, n=4) in isolated Langendorff-perfused rabbit hearts stimulated of 3.5 Hz during 25 minutes of global ischaemia. Until 19 minutes of global ischaemia no significant changes between the two curves exist. Thereafter $[K^+]_0$ was significantly ($p<0.05$) lower in the presence of cromakalim. Data are given as mean ± SD. (Reproduced with permission from A.A.M. Wilde, Cardiovasc Drugs Ther 1993; 7: 521-526.)

However, as shown in Figure 1, KCOs have no effect on the rate of rise of extracellular K^+ concentration during the first 10 minutes of ischaemia (31,39,40,41) This suggests that opening of K_{ATP} channels is not responsible for the net loss of potassium ions from ischaemic cells during the early phase of ischaemia (42).

K_{ATP} channels become more sensitive to KCOs when ATP levels decrease (9,10,43). Therefore, electrophysiologic alterations in ischaemic myocardium may occur at doses of KCOs that have no electrophysiological effects in normoxic tissue. Thus, in ischaemic myocardium, KCOs enhance the rate of action potential shortening (40,44,45,46,47) and this could predispose to re-entry.

It is important to realize that in addition to factors that alter wavelength, a great many factors determine whether arrhythmias occur in the setting of acute ischaemia (31,32). Among the factors are the size of the ischaemic area, which is dependent on the location of the coronary artery occlusion and on the number of pre-existing collaterals; heart rate; nature of anaesthetic agent used or whether any has been used at all; presence of a previous infarction or hypertrophy; the activity of the autonomic nervous system; the number of successive coronary artery occlusions. For example, when pre-existing collaterals are absent, occlusion of the circumflex coronary artery in the canine heart will always cause ventricular fibrillation; when collaterals are abundant, this arrhythmia may never occur (48). It is therefore not surprising that in most studies on the effects of anti-arrhythmic drugs during acute ischaemia, the incidence of arrhythmias in the control group varies widely (49). Trolese-Mongheal and co-workers (49) studied 658 untreated dogs. They found that the sudden death rate following occlusion of the left anterior descending coronary artery varied from 0 to 70% when a series of 10 dogs were used, from 5 to 55% for a series of 20 dogs and from 14 to 36% for a series of 100 dogs. In studies on anti- or pro-arrhythmic effects of drugs during acute ischaemia, ideally, at least the following parameters should be controlled or if not controlled, at least taken into account: size of the ischaemic area, degree of collateral flow, heart rate, level of anaesthesia (or in conscious animals, level of stress), neural input to the heart, and especially for small hearts, the gaseous environment. *When these factors are not considered, studies involving small numbers of dogs must be regarded with caution.*

In the study of Chi et al. (50) dogs with a previous anterior myocardial infarction were subjected to occlusion of the circumflex branch. Of 15 control animals, one dog developed ventricular fibrillation during the first hour following coronary occlusion, against 9 out of 15 dogs treated with pinacidil. It is not clear whether the animals died during the IA or IB phase and no measurements of relevant electrophysiological pacemakers, e.g. action potential duration or refractory period duration, were made. The pinacidil-treated animals had a higher heart rate, suggesting an increased sympathetic tone. Size of the ischaemic zone was unknown, but infarct size was greater in the treatment group than in the control animals. The higher heart rate, the increased sympathetic tone and the larger infarct size will in themselves lead to a higher incidence of arrhythmias. In another dog study, KCOs also appeared to increase the incidence of lethal arrhythmias, although the effect did not reach significance (51), and in a third study no pro-arrhythmic effects were reported (52).

In a recent study, two KCOs, pinacidil and cromakalim, were tested in a pig model, where ventricular fibrillation was reproducibly induced by rapid ventricular pacing following occlusion of the left anterior descending coronary artery, with a relatively constant time to fibrillation (53). Although both compounds produced a similar fall in blood pressure, their electrophysiological effects differed: cromakalim only caused a slight shortening of action potential duration and effective refractory period (7 and 8% respectively) and had no effect on the time to ventricular fibrillation, whereas pinacidil reduced action potential duration and the refractory period by 19% and 16% respectively, and prolonged the time to fibrillation from 134 $\pm$ 5 to 322 $\pm$ 62 sec. In this study, the *antifibrillatory* effect was related to action potential shortening and the authors speculated that this was due to prevention of calcium overload. The results of this study are difficult to interpret. The authors thought that their model produced non-re-entrant arrhythmias (which because of their timing are IA arrhythmias) caused by calcium overload. However, it has been shown that the IA arrhythmias (2 to 10 minutes after the onset of ischaemia) are due to re-entry (see 31,32). The IB arrhythmias, which in the pig occur between 16 and 25 minutes, could very well be related to calcium overload since they occur at the time when cell-to-cell electrical uncoupling develops (54) a process thought to be due to calcium overload.

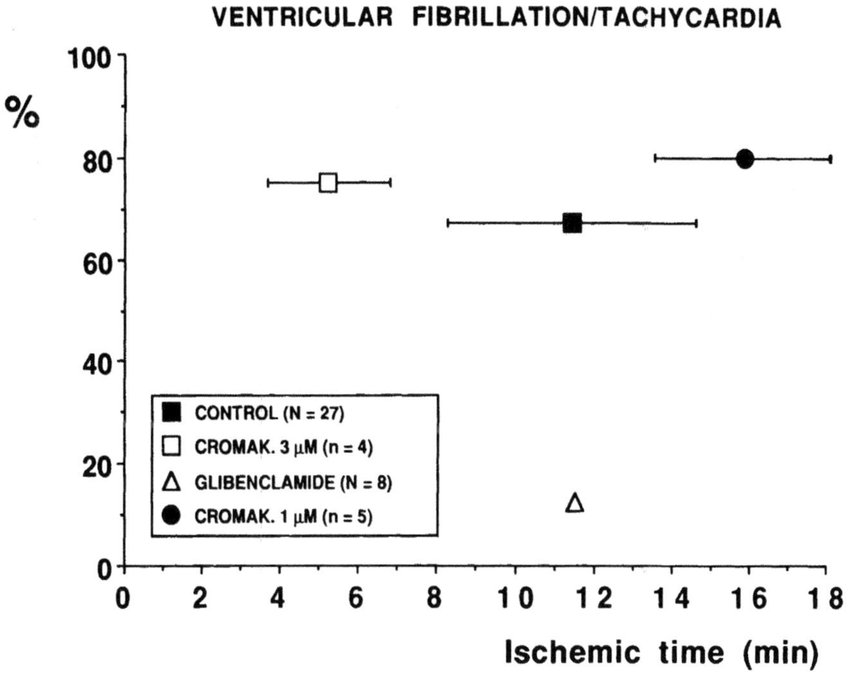

Figure 2. The incidence of ventricular fibrillation and ventricular tachycardia (y-axis) during 16 minutes of global ischaemia in the isolated rabbit heart, stimulated at 3.5 Hz. Glibenclamide (3 mM) markedly reduced the incidence of arrhythmias (open triangle; 1 out of 8 hearts developed VF), whilst the time of occurrence is similar to that in untreated hearts (filled squares = mean time of occurrence ± SD; 18 out of 27 hearts developed VT or VF). In the presence of cromakalim, the incidence of arrhythmias was similar to that in untreated hearts, but the higher dose (3 mM) accelerated the time of onset, the lower dose (1 mM) postponed it. (Modified from A.A.M. Wilde, Cardiovasc Drugs Ther 1993; 7: 521-526.)

Controversial results regarding pro - or anti-arrhythmic effects of KCOs have also been obtained in smaller animals. Our own results during global ischaemia in the isolated Langendorff-perfused rabbit heart (38) are shown in Figure 2. Cromakalim in a dose of 3 uM shortens the time to fibrillation, and prolongs it in a dose of 1 uM. The overall incidence of arrhythmias was similar in all groups. The higher dose of cromakalim, which shortened the QT interval to a greater extent than the low dose, appeared to induce IA arrhythmias in a model that under control conditions only exhibits IB arrhythmias.

That the low dosis of cromakalim prolongs the time to onset of IB arrhythmias is in agreement with the postponement of electrical cell-to-cell uncoupling by this drug (46). In a low-flow ischaemia model in the rat heart, the time to onset of ventricular fibrillation was also shortened by KCOs, but the incidence of fibrillation remained the same as in the control group (55). In an in vivo rat model with a 5 minute occlusion of the left anterior descending coronary artery in which the control animals showed no IA arrhythmias, these arrhythmias did occur in 5 of 14 pinacidil-treated animals (56). However, as in the dog study mentioned earlier (50) heart rate was significantly higher in the treated group. In another study on rats with regional ischaemia, pinacidil and cromakalim in doses which caused only slight changes in heart rate, were actually anti-arrhythmic (57). A possible explanation for these apparently contradictory results is that KCOs during ischaemia may be anti-arrhythmic by virtue of their anti-ischaemic effects and pro-arrhythmic because of marked shortening of the action potential. It is in this respect noteworthy that Yao and Gross (58) recently reported that bimakalim in a dose of 0.1 ug/min did not have an effect on the duration of the monophasic action potential in anaesthetised dogs during acute ischaemia, and did not cause more ventricular fibrillation compared to a control group. It did, however, markedly reduce infarct size. A dose of 0.3 ug/min did accelerate the rate of action potential shortening during ischaemia, but was not arrhythmogenic. Only at a dose of 3.0 ug/min was the incidence of ventricular fibrillation significantly increased. It may therefore be proposed that KCOs at low doses have no effect on IA arrhythmias because they have no, or only minor, effects on action potential duration, and delay the onset of IB arrhythmias. At higher doses they may induce IA arrhythmias in species that normally only exhibit IB arrhythmias, or increase the incidence of such arrhythmias in species that normally do develop them. There clearly is a need for further experimental studies in a well defined animal model of acute ischaemia, with control of heart rate, collateral flow and blood pressure, in which at various doses not only the incidence and timing of IA and IB arrhythmias are studied, but relevant parameters such as action potential duration in and outside the ischaemic zone, time course of development of electrical uncoupling or increase in intracellular calcium concentration, are measured as well.

CONCLUSION

In summary KCOs suppress the arrhythmias during the subacute phase of myocardial infarction, beginning several hours after the onset of ischemia, because they are caused by abnormal automaticity. During the acute phase of ischemia, i.e. the first 30 minutes following acute coronary artery obstruction, KCOs may be both pro and anti-arrhythmic. In the 1A phase (2-10 minutes) accentuated action potential shortening may promote re-entrant arrhythmias; in the 1B phase KCOs may delay the occurrence of arrhythmias by delaying electrical cell-to-cell uncoupling.

REFERENCES

[1] Rensma PL, Allessie MA, Lammers WJEP, Bonke FIM, Schalij MJ. Length of excitation wave and susceptibility to reentrant atrial arrhythmias in normal conscious dogs. Circ Res 1988;62:395-410.

[2] Coussaye JE de la, Eledjam JJ, Bruelle P et al. Electrophysiologic and arrhythmogenic effects of the potassium channel agonist BRL 38227 in anesthetized dogs. J Cardiovasc Pharmacol 1993;22:722-30.

[3] Spinelli W, Follmer C, Parsons R, Colatsky T. Effects of cromakalim, pinacidil and nicorandil on cardiac refractoriness and arterial pressure in open chest dogs. Eur J Pharmacol 1990;179:243-52.

[4] Kojima S, Ishikawa S, Ohsawa K, Mori H. Determination of effective and safe dose for intracoronary administration of nicorandil in dogs. Cardiovasc Res 1990;24:727-32.

[5] Bazil MK, Ukropec JA, Williams PD. Hemodynamic and electrocardiographic (ECG) effects of CL 188,294, a potassium channel opener, in conscious dogs (abstract). Pharmacologist 1993;35:178.

[6] Padrini R, Bova S, Cargnelli G et al. Effects of pinacidil on guinea-pig isolated perfused heart with particular reference to the pro-arrhythmic effect. Br J Pharmacol 1992;105:715-9.

[7] Frydman AM, Chapelle Ph, Diekmann HW et al. Pharmacokinetics of nicorandil. Am J Cardiol 1989;63 (Supp J):25J-33J.

[8] Friedel HA, Brogden RV. Pinacidil. A review of its pharmacodynamic and pharmacokinetic properties, and therapeutic potential in the treatment of hypertension. Drugs 1990;39:929-67.

[9] Hakayama K, Fan Z, Marumo F et al. Action of nicorandil on ATP-sensitive K^+ channel in guinea pig ventricular myocytes. Br J Pharmacol 1991;103: 1641-8.

[10] Arena JP, Kass RS. Enhancement of potassium-sensitive current in heart cells by pinacidil. Circ Res 1989;65:436-45.

[11] Nakayama K, Fan Z, Maruno F, Hiraoka M. Interrelation between pinacidil and intracellular ATP-sensitive K^+ current in guinea pig ventricular myocytes. Circ Res 1990;67:1124-33.

[12] Imanishi S, Arita M, Aomine M, Kiyosue T. Antiarrhythmic effects of nicorandil on canine cardiac Purkinje fibers. J Cardiovasc Pharmacol 1984; 6:772-9.

[13] De Diego JM, Antzelevitch C. Pinacidil-included electrical heterogeneity and extrasystolic activity in canine ventricular tissue. Circulation 1993; 88:1177-89.

[14] Goldberg MR. Clinical pharmacology of pinacidil, a prototype for drugs that affect potassium channel. J Cardiovasc Pharmacol 1988;12(Suppl 2):S41-S47.

[15] Nony P. Girard P, Arnand P et al. Electrophysiologic effects of a potassium channel activator (pinacidil) on repolarization parameters in healthy volunteers: a surface ECG study. J Cardiovasc Pharmacol 1993;22:534-9.

[16] Krumenacker M, Roland E. Clinical profile of nicorandil, an overview of its hemodynamic properties and therapeutic efficacy. J Cardiovasc Pharmacol 1992;20 (Suppl III):S94-S102.

[17] Liu B, Golyan F, McCullough JR, Vassalle M. Electrophysiological and antiarrhythmic effect of the K-channel opener, BRL 34915, in cardiac Purkinje fibers. Drug Dev Res 1988;14:123-39.

[18] Lathrop DA, Nanasi PP, Varro A. In vitro cardiac models of dog Purkinje fibre triggered and spontaneous electrical activity: effects of nicorandil. Br J Pharmacol 1990;99:114-23.

[19] Spinelli W, Sorota S, Siegal M, Hoffman BF. Antiarrhythmic actions of the ATP-regulated K^+ current activated by pinacidil. Circ Res 1991;68:1127-37.

[20] Gotanda K, Satoh K, Taira N. Is the cardiovascular profile of BRL 34915 characteristic of potassium channel activators? J Cardiovasc Pharmacol 1998;12:239-46.

[21] Task Force of the Working Group on Arrhythmias of the European Society of Cardiology. The Sicilian Gambit. A new approach to the classification of antiarrhythmic drugs based on their action on arrhythmogenic mechanisms. Circulation 1991;84:1831-51, and Eur Heart J 1991;12:1112-31.

[22] Members of the Sicilian Gambit. Antiarrhythmic Therapy: a pathophysiological approach. Armonk NY: Futura Publishing Company Inc, 1994.

[23] Kerr MJ, Wilson R, Shanks RG. Suppression of ventricular arrhythmias after coronary artery ligation by pinacidil, a vasodilator drug. J Cardiovasc Pharmacol 1985;7:875-83.

[24] Komori S, Ishii M, Hashimoto K. Antiarrhythmic effects of coronary vasodilators on canine ventricular arrhythmia models. Jpn J Pharmacol 1985;38:73-82.

[25] Hashimoto K, Haruno A, Matsuzaki T et al. Effects of antiarrhythmic drugs on canine ventricular arrhythmia models: which electrophysiological characteristics of drugs are related to their effectivenss? Cardiovasc Drugs Ther 1991;5:805-18.

[26] Fish FA, Prakash C, Roden DM. Suppression of repolarization related arrhythmias in vitro and in vivo by low-dose potassium channel activator. Circulation 1990;82:1362-9.

[27] Takahashi N, Ito M, Saikawa T, Arita M. Nicorandil suppressess early afterdepolarizations and ventricular arrhythmias induced by ceasium chloride in rabbits in vivo. Cardiovasc Res 1991;25:445-452.

[28] Vos MA, de Groot M, Lipcsei GE et al. Lemakalim demonstrates mechanism of specific antiarrhythmic properties without proarrhythmogenity (abstract). Circulation 1992;86(Suppl I):I-560.

[29] Carlsson L, Abrahamsson C, Drews L, Duker G. Antiarrhythmic effect of potassium channel openers in rhythm abnormalities related to delayed repolarization. Circulation 1992;85:1491-500.

[30] D'Alonzo AJ, Hess TA, Darbenzio RB, Sewter JC. Effects of intracoronary cromakalim, pinacidil, or diltiazem on cesium-chloride-induced arrhythmias in anesthetized dogs under conditions of controlled coronary blood flow. J Cardiovasc Pharmacol 1993;21:677-83.

[31] Janse MJ, Wit AL. Electrophysiological mechanisms of ventricular arrhythmias resulting from myocardial ischemia and infarction. Physiol Rev 1989;69:1049-169.

[32] Wit AL, Janse MJ. The ventricular arrhythmias of ischemia and infarction. Electrophysiological mechanisms. Mount Kisco NY, Futura Publishing Company Inc, 1993.

[33] Daugherty A, Frayne KN, Redfern WS, Woodward B. The role of catechol-amines in the production of ischemia-induced ventricular arrhythmias in the rat in vivo and in vitro. Br J Pharmacol 1986;87:265-77.

[34] Penny WJ. The deleterious effects of myocardial catecholamines on cellular electrophysiology and arrhythmias during ischemia and reperfusion. Eur Heart J 1984;5:960-73.

[35] Corr PB, Witkowski FX, Sobel BE. Mechanisms contributing to malignant arrhythmias induced by ischemia in the cat. J Clin Invest 1978;61:109-119.

[36] Cotor SJ. Anesthetized rabbit as a model for ischemia- and reperfusion-induced arrhythmias. J Pharmacol Methods 1989;21:263-79.

[37] Coronel R, Wilms-Schopman FJG, Dekker LRC, Janse, MJ. Heterogeneities in $[K^+]_o$ and TQ potential, and the inducibility by ventricular fibrillation during acute regional ischemia in the isolated perfused porcine heart. Circulation 1995 (in press).

[38] Wilde AAM. Role of ATP-sensitive K^+ channel current in ischemic arrhythmias. Cardiovasc Drugs Ther 1993;7:521-6.

[39] Mitani A, Kinoshita K, Fukamachi K et al. Effects of glibenclamide and nicorandil on cardiac function during ischemia and reperfusion. Am J Physiol 1991;261:H1864-H71.

[40] Venkatesh N, Stuart JS, Lamp ST, Alexander LD, Weiss JN. Activation of ATP-sensitive K^+ channels by cromakalim. Effects of cellular K^+ loss and cardiac function in ischemic and reperfused mammalian ventricle. Circ Res 1992;71:1324-33.

[41] Vanheel B, de Hemptinne A. Influence of K_{ATP} channel modulation on net potassium efflux from ischaemic mammalian cardiac tissue. Cardiovasc Res 1992;26:1030-9.

[42] Wilde AAM, Aksnes, G. Myocardial potassium loss and cell depolarisation in ischaemia and hypoxia. Cardiovasc res 1995;29:1-15.

[43] Martin CL, Chinn K. Pinacidil opens ATP-dependent K^+ channels in an ATP- and temperature-dependent manner. J Cardiovasc Pharmacol 1990;15:510-4.

[44] Cole WC, McPherson CD, Sontag D. ATP regulated K^+ channels protect the myocardium against ischemia/reperfusion damage. Circ Res 1991;69:571-81.

[45] Wilde AAM, Schumacher CA, Fiolet JWT et al. Opening of ATP-sensitive potassium channel does not necessarily contribute to potassium accumulation in the globally ischemic rabbit heart (abstract). J Mol Cell Cardiol 1992;24:S276.

[46] Tan HL, Mazón P, Verberne HJ et al. Ischaemic preconditioning delays ischaemia-induced cellular uncoupling by activation of ATP sensitive potassium channels. Cardiovasc Res 1993;27:644-51.

[47] D'Alonzo AJ, Darbenzio RB, Parham CS, Grover GJ. Effects of intracoronary cromakalim on postischaemic contractile function and action potential duration. Cardiovasc Res 1992;26:1046-53

[48] Meesmann W. Early arrhythmias and primary ventricular fibrillation after acute myocardial ischaemia in relation to pre-existing coronary collaterals. In: Early arrhythmias resulting from myocardial ischaemia. Mechanisms and prevention by drugs. JR Parratt (ed), London, MacMillan, 1982; 93-112.

[49] Trolese-Mongheal Y, Duchene-Marullaz P, Trolese JF et al. Sudden death and experimental acute myocardial infarction. Am J Cardiol 1985;56:677-81.

[50] Chi L, Uprichard ACG, Lucchesi BR. Profibrillatory actions of pinacidil in a conscious canine model of sudden coronary death. J Cardiovasc Pharmacol 1990;15:452-64.

[51] Kitzen JM, McCallum JD, Harvey C et al. Potassium channel activators cromakalim and celikalim (WAY-120,491) fail to decrease myocardial infarct size in the anesthetized canine. Pharmacology 1992;45:71-82.

[52] Grover GJ, Dzwonczyk S, Parham CS, Sleph PG. The protective effects of cromakalim and pinacidil on reperfusion function and infarct size in isolated perfused rat hearts and anesthetized dogs. Cardiovasc Drugs Ther 1990;4:465-74.

[53] D'Alonzo AJ, Hess TA, Darbenzio RB et al. Effects of cromakalim or pinacidil on pacing- and ischaemia-induced ventricular fibrillation in the anesthetized pig. Basic Res Cardiol 1994;89:162-76.

[54] Smith WT, Fleet WF, Johnson TA, Cascio WE. The I-B phase of ventricular arrhythmias in ischemic in situ porcine heart is related to changes in cell-to-cell electrical coupling (abstract). Circulation 1994;90:I-524.

[55] Wolleben CD, Sanguinetti MC, Siegl PKS. Influence of ATP-sensitive potassium modulators on ischemia-induced fibrillation in isolated rat hearts. J Mol Cell Cardiol 1989;21:783-788.

[56] Lu H, Remeysen O, De Clerc F. The protection by ischemic preconditioning against myocardial ischemia- and reperfusion-induced arrhythmias is not mediated by ATP-sensitive potassium channels in the rat. Cor Art Dis 1993;4:649-57.

[57] D'Alonzo AJ, Darbenzio RB, Hess TA et al. Effect of potassium on the action of the K_{ATP} modulators cromakalim, pinacidil, or glibenclamide on arrhythmias in isolated perfused rat heart subjected to regional ischaemia. Cardiovasc Res 1994;28:881-7.

[58] Yao Z, Gross GJ. Effects of the K_{ATP} channel opener bimakalim on coronary blood flow, monophasic action potential duration, and infarct size in dogs. Circulation 1994;89:1769-75.

6

CLINICAL EXPLOITATION OF THE K_{ATP} CHANNEL

HENRY PURCELL and KIM FOX

The Royal Brompton Hospital, Sydney Street, London SW3 6NP, UK.

INTRODUCTION

Potassium ion (K^+) channels play a dominant role in controlling the resting membrane potential of excitable cells. They are ubiquitous, structurally diverse and functionally are perhaps most usefully classified by what causes them to open or close. Receptor-activated channels are influenced, either directly or indirectly, via messengers notably adenosine triphosphate (ATP). Activation of the so-called ATP-sensitive K+ channels (K_{ATP}) is inhibited (closed) at physiological levels of intracellular ATP and open when the intracellular ATP concentration falls. These ATP-sensitive K+ channels also act as membrane receptor sites for various drugs. The enormously increased interest in K+ channel inhibitors and openers (KCOs) suggests that these ion channels are rife for clinical exploitation. This review is not intended to be exhaustive but will focus selectively on the development and therapeutic potential of these pharmacological modulators in cardiovascular disease.

While workers continue to explore the molecular biology of the K_{ATP} channel (2), much has been learned from observations using 'first generation' K+ channel opening (KCO) compounds. These include cromakalim, diazoxide and minoxidil, and agents which antagonise their effects, probably specifically (3), such as the sulphonylureas, tolbutamide and glibenclamide which are used in the treatment of diabetes (4). Other drugs including the antiarrhythmics sotalol and amiodarone probably block the K+ channel non-specifically. K+ channel openers acting on KATP channels have been divided into seven structural classes (5) these structural types together with prototypes in each class are shown in Table 1.

Table 1. Potassium channel openers; classification of synthetic agents

Structural type	**Prototype**
Benzopyrans	levcromakalim
Thioureas/cyanoguanidines	pinacidil
Pyridines	nicorandil
Pyrimidines/triazines	minoxidil
Benzothiadiazines	diazoxide
Thioformamides	aprikalim
Dihydropyridines	niguldipine

The large number of these compounds in development reflects the immense interest and efforts invested in synthesising new drugs intended to circumvent the limitations of the 'first-generation' agents of this class.

The principal classes under active research are the benzopyrans, the thioureas/cyanoguanidines, the thioformamides and the pyridine derivatives. A summary of 'lead compounds' and their development status is shown in Appendix 1. Because of the lack of selectivity of first-generation compounds, which as one author describes, open K_{ATP} channels in a "promiscuous manner" (6), newer drugs are more likely to be tissue-selective and therefore have greater therapeutic potential. The prime target of KCOs has been vascular smooth muscle where they can induce vasodilatation and a reduction in systemic vascular resistance (7,8). They are now also considered candidates for use in a variety of cardiovascular disorders, chronic obstructive airways disease and diverse conditions including irritable bladder and impotence. Many of the potential indications claimed in patent applications are speculative and based on their in vitro pharmacology which is not yet supported by clinical data. Some currently available and investigational K+ channel modulators are outlined in Table 2. There are at least 62 pharmaceutical companies active in this field, including SmithKline Beecham, which has secured patents on at least 25 K^+ channel modulators, and is the leading research company in this field.

Table 2. Pharmaceutical companies identified as being active in K+ channel modulator research and development

Companies active in potassium channel modulator research

COMPANY	MODULAR TYPE	LEAD COMPOUND
Adir	A	-
Alkaloida	A	-
Almirall	A	-
American Home Products	A	celikalim, WAY 120, 129
	B	risotilide
BASF	B	-
Beiersdorf	A	BDF 9333
Bristol-Myers Squibb	B	*d*-sotalol
Boehringer Ingelheim	B	zatebradine, alinidine
Chugai	A	(nicorandil)
Ciba Geigy	A	CGP 42500
Eastman (Sterling)	B	(gliquidone)
Eisai	A	E4080
	B	E4031
Eli Lilly	A	LY 211808, LY 206300
E. Merck	A	bimakalim, emakalim
Fujisawa	A	FR 119748
Green Cross	A	AL - 0671
Hoechst	A	Hoe234, SO121
	B	(glibenclamide, tolbutamide)
Hoffman La Roche	A	Ro 31-6930
ICI	B	-
Interneuron	B	-
ISIS Innovation	B	-
Kaken	A	KP-294
Johnson & Johnson	A	RWJ 29009
Kanebo	A	-
Kirin	A	KRN2391
Leo	A	(pinacidil) P1060
Lonza	A	-
Merck	B	L-691,121, L-702,958, L-706,000
Mochida	B	5-HD, M14157
Nepera	A	-
Nissan	A	NIP 121
Nycomed (Hafslund)	A	
Pfizer	A	
	B	dofetilide, UK 66914
Pola Chemical	A	LP-805
Procter & Gamble	A	NE-10064
Rhone Poulenc Rorer	A	aprikalim
	B	terikalant
Sandoz	A	SDZ PCO 400
Sanofi	A	SR 47063
Schering AG (Berlex)	B	sematilide
Servier	B	(glicazide)
SmithKline Beecham	A	levcromakalim, BRL 55834
Solvay (Kali Chemie)	B	tedisamil
Syntex	A	-
Takeda		TCV-295
Upjohn	A	(minoxidil), ibutilide
Uriach	A	-
Yamanouchi	A	YM934, YM099
Yoshitomi	A	Y27152

A denotes K+ channel activator (opener) while B denotes K+ channel blocker (inhibitor). Table reproduced by kind permission of Current Drugs Ltd.

FIRST GENERATION K^+ CHANNEL OPENERS

The cardiovascular and biological effects of prototype K^+ openers and inhibitors have been extensively reviewed (9,10). These include marketed antihypertensive drugs such as diazoxide, minoxidil and pinacidil. Diazoxide acts on the K^+ channels of pancreatic B-cells which modulate insulin secretion. Hyperglycaemia is a common effect due to inhibition of insulin release, an action which can be turned to good effect in the management of chronic hypoglycaemia. Its use in hypertension is restricted to hypertensive emergencies however, when it may be given as a rapid bolus injection, or more cautiously in a series of small boluses or as an intravenous infusion, to lower blood pressure acutely. Diazoxide may cause frank hypotension and it may also induce reflex tachycardia. It should not be used in patients with dissecting aortic aneurysm. Side-effects of this drug are well-documented and include sodium and fluid retention, hyperuricaemia, hyperglycaemia and hyperlipidaemia (11). Its use should therefore be restricted to short-term emergency treatment and other agents may be preferable.

Minoxidil also has some use orally in hypertensive urgencies and emergencies, as well as in severe hypertension in conjunction with other antihypertensives. Sodium and water retention also occur with minoxidil while weight gain, peripheral oedema and tachycardia (which may precipitate angina) may be troublesome. For unexplained reasons minoxidil causes hypertrichosis in 80% of patients after 3-6 weeks therapy (11); this effect has been used in the treatment of alopecia. Minoxidil is marketed in the UK as Regaine (Upjohn) a hair restorer.

Pinacidil, although not available in the UK is used in other countries for management of patients with mild to moderate essential hypertension and secondary renal hypertension. In clinical trials pinacidil has been shown to be as effective as hydralazine, prazosin and nifedipine in achieving blood pressure control. Despite acting as a KCO, pinacidil causes adverse effects typical of peripheral vasodilators (12) and oedema, headache, dizziness and palpitations are commonly reported, while hypertrichosis is less common than that observed with minoxidil. A recent study of 257 hypertensive patients (13) compared efficacy and quality of life between pinacidil (up to 100 mg daily) and nifedipine (20-80 mg daily), with background diuretic therapy. Goal blood pressure was achieved similarly with both drugs and overall patients tended to have fewer complaints at the end of the trial compared to entry. Complaints of growth of body and facial hair were noted in the pinacidil group, but there were no significant differences with respect to other side-effects. Notably, in assessments of psychological well-being, pinacidil-treated patients showed a significant improvement in total and cognitive function scores compared to nifedipine.

Electrocardiographic T-wave changes, reflecting abnormal repolarization, have been observed in 30% of patients treated with pinacidil and patients have also reported palpitations and tachycardia (14). Such observations are regarded as cause for concern and underline important reservations on the clinical use of the KCO class in treatment of hypertension and arrhythmia, particularly in those postinfarction patients who are known to be at high risk of sudden death (15). Chi and co-workers (16) have investigated the effects of pinacidil and the K_{ATP} inhibitor, glibenclamide in an isolated rabbit heart model and findings suggest that under conditions of hypoxia (decrease in myocardial ATP concentration) and reoxygenation, pinacidil may facilitate the development of ventricular fibrillation, an effect which can be reduced by glibenclamide.

Wilde (17) argues that such evidence should be regarded with caution, and that KCOs are only arrhythmogenic in the presence of low potassium, as was the case in the hypoxic perfused rabbit model; and that in non-ischaemic conditions KCOs are only proarrhythmic in high, hypotensive "and thus probably irrelevant" doses. It appears therefore that action potential shortening is dose-dependent (3) and while agents such as pinacidil unequivocaly shorten cardiac action potential duration and may promote re-entry, conflicting results on proarrhythmia may be explained on the basis of inappropriate animal models, and the mechanisms of particular arrhythmias. Some comfort may be derived from observations that proarrhythmic KCO-effects have not been observed in man (18). Clinical studies, some of which have involved ambulatory electrocardiographic (Holter) monitoring, have not identified any increase in sudden cardiac deaths or lethal arrhythmia so that they are unlikely to be deleterious at therapeutic doses. The debate as to whether KCOs are likely (19) or unlikely (20) to be proarrhythmic in the diseased human heart is far from resolved, and more data are needed from relevant animal models and clinical trials.

NEWER AGENTS

The profound hypotensive effect induced by some KCOs has led to further disquiet about their use in the clincal setting. It was therefore hoped that compounds such as BMS-180448, which possess anti-ischaemic but little or no smooth muscle relaxant activity (6) might provide useful anti-anginal properties without compromising haemodynamic variables. Regretably, BMS-180448 will not be taken to registration because of elevated liver enzyme levels which were seen in several patients after prolonged treatment (GJ Grover, personal communication). Interest remains in other KCOs which may possess minimal hypotensive effects and also in the new class of sinus-node inhibitors, which reduce heart rate and myocardial oxygen demand, but unlike beta blockers, do not lower blood pressure.

Clearly, efficient blood pressure lowering is desirable in the development of new antihypertensive therapy, and the benzopyran derivative, cromakalim (formerly BRL 34915) which might be regarded as the prototype of the specific KCOs (21), is a vasodilator with potent hypotensive properties (22). Cromakalim
development has ceased and clinical work has has been conducted using the active enantiomer levcromakalim which may also possess antiarrhythmic effects (23). Initially levcromakalim was under active development as an anti-asthmatic and antihypertensive, but it is no longer of interest as a respiratory agent. In the UK it is currently in phase 3 trials as an antihypertensive, and a patent application has been filed for levcromakalim as a hypolipidaemic. It is suggested that given the right dose, to minimize problems of reflex tachycardia and headache, "it may find a niche" (24). Other novel agents which combine KCO and angiotensin 11-receptor antagonist activity are also currently in early development for treatment of angina and hypertension.

FIRST GENERATION K^+ CHANNEL BLOCKERS

In most cells the intracellular ATP concentration is probably sufficient to ensure that the KATP channel is usually closed under normal conditions. In the pancreatic B-cell, intracellular ATP appears to be subject to marked fluctuations, and increases as plasma glucose increases (25). The resulting closure of KATP channels depolarises the beta-cell, increasing calcium ion influx, and triggers insulin release. Oral hypoglycaemic agents such as glibenclamide inhibit K_{ATP} channels which results in an increase in insulin release. Studies conducted by Wallner and co-workers on the effects of sulphonylureas on hypoxia and ischaemia-induced coronary vasodilatation in isolated Langendorff-perfused guinea pig hearts, suggest that sulphonylureas may prevent the vital coronary response to ischaemia, ie local vasodilatation and mobilisation of coronary reserve. This might account for the increased cardiovascular mortality reported during the last 20 years in patients treated with these compounds (26). The antagonistic effect of glibenclamide on the K_{ATP} channel has, however provided a unique pharmacological tool and a rapid 'on-the-spot' test (27) to study the profiles of vasorelaxant drugs which may be suspected to work predominantly via K^+ channel modulation.

Many structurally-diverse agents are now classified as K^+ channel blockers or inhibitors. These range from naturally-occurring toxins to synthetic agents such as the sulphonylureas. Clinically the use of these agents falls into three categories (28);

1) Non-insulin dependent diabetes mellitus eg glibenclamide, meglitinide
2) Antiarrhythmic agents (Class 111 type) eg sematilide, dofetilide
3) Sinus node inhibitors (bradycardic agents) eg tedisamil, Zeneca D7288, zatebradine

A considerable degree of attention is now focussed on drugs which prolong the cardiac action potential, and refractory period, ie class 111 antiarrhythmic agents. Such agents, by causing QT-interval prolongation are also potentially proarrhythmic especially in hypokalaemic individuals (29). However, as they may not cause significant blood pressure changes or cardiodepressant effects at clinical doses, they may be useful in ischaemic heart disease.

Classical members of the group include amiodarone and sotalol, which also display other activities. 'Pure' K^+ channel inhibitors are now under clinical evaluation and these are targeted towards voltage-activated channels in cardiac cells (30). These inhibitors include tedisamil, a new bradycardiac agent which has demonstrated antiarrhythymic activity, and favourable haemodynamic and anti-ischaemic effects in rats and primates. It is reported to be well tolerated when given intravenously to patients with coronary artery disease (31), while the most frequent adverse event associated with oral dosing appears to be diarrhoea. The anti-anginal efficacy of tedisamil is currently being assessed in clinical trials.

Dofetilide, another selective class 111, K^+ channel inhibitor has proved effective in animal models and in patients with inducible tachyarrhythmias (32). So far there have been no reports of pro-arrhythmia in man and the incidence of arrhythmias such as torsade de pointes with this agent is as yet unknown. The therapeutic value of the many pure K^+ channel inhibitors which are under development requires further investigation. A new Ca++ / K^+ channel inhibitor, BRL-32872 under development by SmithKline Beecham is in phase 1 trials as an antiarrhythmic (33). The likelihood of torsade de pointes may be reduced with this agent because of its dual mode of action. However, the potential benefits of all of these new agents, must be balanced against the proarrhythmic effects "purportedly associated" with action potential prolongation (30), especially in patients with compromised left ventricular function.

CARDIOPROTECTION

The term cardioprotection is widely used but ill-defined. In the broadest sense it denotes a drug which reduces morbidity and mortality from coronary artery disease (34). Several workers have suggested that KCO drugs may have cardioprotective properties, most notably nicorandil (35), aprikalim (36) and bimakalim (37), following the beneficial effects observed in animal models of ischaemia/reperfusion injury. While such findings may not apply directly to man, we can speculate that K^+ channel openers may to some extent mimic natural cardioprotective processes (38).

Hybrid KCOs

Extensive information is now available on the clinical (39,40) and experimental (41) cardioprotective properties of nicorandil. This is described as a 'hybrid' (42) consisting of a nicotinamide nitrate with KCO activity. The drug was registered in Japan in 1984 for treatment of angina pectoris, and became available for use in the UK and other European countries some ten years later. Nicorandil is an interesting compound for several reasons. Primarily it appears to relieve angina even though it has not been shown as monotherapy to be superior to placebo in all studies of exercise-induced angina (43). The majority of studies demonstrate comparable efficacy to standard agents such as long-acting oral nitrates, beta blockers, propranolol and atenolol, and calcium antagonists including nifedipine and diltiazem. While nicorandil is not a 'pure' K^+ channel opener, it does not behave totally as an organic nitrate and patients do not appear to develop haemodynamic tolerance during continuous intravenous infusion (44).

The KCO activity of nicorandil leads **indirectly** to calcium ion channel blockade, and dilatation of arterial resistance vessels. Furthermore the nitrate moiety activates guanylate cyclase, which increases intracellular cyclic guanosine monophospate (cGMP) causing dilatation of venous capacitance vessels. This novel combination provides a dual mode of action. A recent study has shown that nicorandil is a coronary microvascular dilator (45). An intracoronary bolus of nicorandil rapidly induced maximal coronary hyperaemia comparable to that achieved with intracoronary papaverine.

At therapeutic doses nicorandil has little effect on blood pressure and hypotension is not induced. Similarly, it normally causes minimal increase in heart rate. The most frequently-described side effect with nicorandil is headache, with one long-term study showing an 8.5% drop-out rate related to headache (46). The majority of headaches are experienced in the initial stages of therapy and may be minimized by titrating upwards from a dose of (nicorandil) 5 mg twice daily.

From the clinical experience gained with nicorandil in Japan, along with exercise studies, electrophysiological investigations and Holter monitoring studies in volunteers, nicorandil does not appear to induce arrhythmias when used over its therapeutic dose range (47). The drug is currently being investigated in patients with unstable angina and left ventricular dysfunction. Smaller previously published studies in these areas have not shown nicorandil to be proarrhythmic.

The other principal reason which makes nicorandil an attractive proposition for management of coronary artery disease are its putative cardioprotective properties. Gross and colleagues (41) have conducted experiments showing nicorandil to be "a highly efficacious myocardial protective agent" in several animal models of reversible and irreversible ischaemia-reperfusion injury. In dogs pre-treated with nicorandil, this agent reduced infarct size, expressed as a percent of the area at risk, compared to dogs pre-treated with nifedipine or placebo. Similarly, after a single episode of 10-15 minutes of coronary artery occlusion in dogs, nicorandil administration resulted in enhanced recovery of regional systolic shortening, a measure of contractile function, during reperfusion. During reperfusion-injury neutrophils infiltrate tissue producing super-oxide radicals; nicorandil has been shown to inhibit such neutrophil infiltration. These effects do not appear to be due to its nitrate-like activity, as nitroglycerine was ineffective in this model. The mechanisms underlying these effects are unknown but they may be due to mimicking physiological 'preconditioning' (48), (reviewed elsewhere), which provides powerful protection from ischaemic necrosis.

KCOs are more potent on smooth muscle compared with cardiac cells. Thus therapeutic doses which lead to coronary or systemic vasodilatation have few effects on cardiac myocytes. However, we do not know whether currently-available K^+ channel modulators have greater effects on cardiac K^+ channels under clinical (in vivo) conditions (so that much lower drug concentrations will activate them) (49). Clearly the concept of cardioprotection may become more relevant as new compounds which show greater binding to the myocardium and coronary vasculature, become available.

Additional cardioprotective properties reported for nicorandil include antiplatelet effects characteristic of organic mononitrates (50), and enhanced cardioprotection during hyperkalaemic cardioplegia, as reflected by improved recovery of mechanical function after reoxygenation in guinea pig papillary muscle preparations (51).

KRN2391 is another interesting compound which has KCO activity and a nitrate moiety. It is now in early phase 2 development. KRN2391 is also considered to have a dual mechanism of action and it possesses potent vasodilating properties with some selectivity for the coronary vascular bed. KRN2391 has greater potency and longer duration of action than nicorandil and increases coronary blood flow in a manner similar to nifedipine. In addition, blood pressure was less affected by KRN2391 than was coronary blood flow compared to these other two agents (52).

KRN2391 appears to show more KCO (as opposed to nitrate-like) activity (53), and as with nicorandil, experiments in dogs appear to show that KRN2391 does not induce acute tolerance- as assessed by the effects on coronary blood flow during intracoronary infusion, either by itself or cross-tolerance between KRN2391 and other nitrates (54). In experiments using a perfused rat heart model, both KRN2391 and nicorandil at high doses were shown to have cardioprotective effects on ischaemic dysfunction (55).

Not all KCOs are cardioprotective. Reduction in infarct size and attenuation of myocardial stunning were not observed with the benzopyran derivatives, cromakalim and WAY-120,491 (celikalim) which is no longer in clinical trials (TJ Colatsky, personal communication) in a dog model of ischaemic injury (56). It remains to be seen whether the interesting findings with agents such as bimakalim (57) which protects against ischaemia-related injury in the pig, and is in phase 2 development; and emakalim (EMD 56431) and symakalim (EMD 57283) which are in phase 2 and late preclinical phase respectively (N Beir, personal communication), which have reported anti-ischaemic/antihypertensive potential, will afford benefits in the clinical setting.

CONCLUSION

It might be argued that the clinical thrust of Ca^{++} ion channels and their antagonists has been eclipsed by the current interest in K^{+} channels and compounds which open or close them. Calcium antagonists have however made an enormous contribution to the treatment of angina and hypertension, while the clinical benefits of K^{+} modulators have yet to be realised. There is little dispute that they are rife for clinical exploitation.

The deficiencies in current cardiovascular drug therapy are well recognised. However, for any new drug class to succeed it must be as good as, and preferably better than, existing therapy. So far it has not been possible to demonstrate clear advantages of the K^{+} channel modulators. This problem has been compounded by the typical vasodilator-type side effects observed in earlier generation agents. This may improve with better tissue selectivity, which although not well-understood, seems to be related to the existence of receptor subtypes in different tissues (58). Hopefully the newer drugs in this fascinating and exciting family may provide benefit, especially in the field of cardioprotection. This has so far only been achieved with aspirin and beta blockers in the prevention of myocardial reinfarction.

REFERENCES

1 Cook NS. The pharmacology of potassium channels and their therapeutic modulation. Trends Pharmacol Sci 1988;9:21-28.

2 Nichols CG. Molecular biology of the KATP channel. Where's the clone? Cardiovasc Res 1994;28:727-728.

3 Wilde AAM, Janse MJ. Electrophysiological effects of ATP sensitive potassium channel modulation: implications for arrhythmogenesis. Cardiovasc Res 1994;28:16-24.

4 Edwards G, Weston AH. The pharmacology of ATP-sensitive potassium channels. Ann Rev Pharmacol Toxicol 1993;33:597-637.

5 de Weille JR. Modulation of ATP sensitive potassium channels. Cardiovasc Res 1992;26:1017-1020.

6 Atwal K. Pharmacology and structure-activity relationships for KATP modulators: Tissue-selective KATP openers. J Cardiovasc Pharmacol 1994;24 (suppl 4):S12-S17.

7 Haeusler G. K+-channel openers: New antihypertensive drugs? Clin Physiol Biochem 1990;8 (suppl 2):46-56.

8 Edwards G, Weston AH. Potassium channel openers and vascular smooth muscle relaxation. Pharmac Ther 1990;48:237-258.

9 Richer C, Pratz J, Mulder P, Mondot S, Giudicelli JF, Cavero I. Cardiovascular and biological effects of K+ channel openers, a class of drugs with vasorelaxant and cardioprotective properties. Life Sciences 1990;47:1693-1705

10 Escande D, Henry P. Potassium channels as pharmacological targets in cardiovascular medicine. Eur Heart J 1993;14 (suppl B):2-9.

11 MacCarthy EP. Vasodilators. Chp 10, 183-205. in Hypertension. Eds Punzi HA, Flamenbaum W. Futura Publishing Co Inc, Mount Kisco, New York. 1989.

12 Friedel HA, Brogden RN. Pinacidil; a review of its pharmacodynamic and pharmacokinetic properties, and therapeutic potential in the treatment of hypertension. Drugs 1990;39(6):929-967.

13 Fletcher AE, Battersby C, Adnitt et al. Quality of life on antihypertensive therapy: A double-blind trial comparing quality of life on pinacidil and nifedipine in combination with a thiazide diuretic. J Cardiovasc Pharmacol 1992;20:108-114.

14 Goldberg MR. Clinical pharmacology of pinacidil, a prototype for drugs that affect potassium channels. J Cardiovasc Pharmacol 1988;12(suppl 2):S30-40.

15 Tosaki A, Hellegouarch A. Adenosine triphosphate-sensitive potassium channel blocking agent ameliorates, but the opening agent aggravates, ischemia/reperfusion-induced injury. Heart function studies in nonfibrillating isolated hearts. J Am Coll Cardiol 1994;23:487-96.

16 Chi L, Black SC, Kuo PI, Fagbemi SO, Lucchesi BR. Actions of pinacidil at a reduced potassium concentration: a direct cardiac effect possibly involving the ATP-dependent potassium channel. J Cardiovasc Pharmacol 1993;21:179-190.

17 AAM Wilde. Proarrhythmic potential of potassium channel openers. Cardiovasc Res 1994;28:928-929.

18 Colatsky TJ, Follmer CH. K+ channel blockers and activators in cardiac arrhythmias. Cardiovasc Drug Rev 1989;7:199-209.

19 Black SC, Lucchesi BR. Potassium channel openers are likely to be proarrhythmic in the diseased human heart. Cardiovasc Res 1994;28:923-924.

20 D'Alonzo AJ, Grover GJ. Potassium channel openers are unlikely to be proarrhythmic in the diseased human heart. Cardiovasc Res 1994;28:925.

21 Richer C, Pratz J, Mulder P, Mondot S, Giudicelli JF, Cavero I. Cardiovascular and biological effects of K+ channel openers, a class of drugs with vasorelaxant and cardioprotective properties. Life Sciences 1990;47:1693-1705.

22 Vandenburg MJ, Woodward SR, Hossain M, Stewart-Long P, Tasker TCG. Potassium channel activators lower blood pressure: An initial study of BRL 34915 in hypertensive patients. J Hypertens 1986;4 (suppl 6):S166-S167.

23 Vos M, Gorgels A, Leunissen H, Lipcsei G, de Groot S, Wellens HJJ. Specific anti-arrhythmic effects of the I K-activator lemakalim in vivo. Eur Heart J 1992;13: (Abstract Suppl):61.

24 Anonymous. Lead compound factfile;levcromakalim. in Potassium channel modulators handbook. SMI 1-17 Current Drugs Ltd, London April 1994.

25 Edwards G, Weston A. Potassium channels- what are they and why should we open them? Br J Cardiol 1995;2:43-46.

26 Wallner M, Gasser R, Grisold M, Eber B, Brussee H, Klein W. Increased cardiovascular mortality under sulfonylurea treatment in patients with coronary artery disease:involvement of K+ATP-channels? Eur Heart J 1994;15 (Abstract suppl):506.

27 Kreye VAW, Lenz T, Pfrunder D. Mode of action of potassium channel openers in vascular smooth muscle. Rev Contemp Pharmacother 1993;4:185-198.

28 Weston AH. Ion channels as targets for drugs. (Abstract) Presentation to The Society for Drug Research; Potassium channel modulators- new therapeutic opportunities, Meeting, London, 9 March 1993.

29 Singh BN, Opie LH, Harrison DC, Marcus FI. Antiarrhythmic agents. chp 4, pp 54-90. in Drugs for the heart, Opie LH, ed. 2nd edition. Grune & Stratton Inc, Orlando. 1987

30 Escande D, Henry P. Potassium channels as pharmacological targets in cardiovascular medicine. Eur Heart J 1993;14 (suppl B):2-9.

31 Mitrovic V, Oehm E, Liebrich A, Thormann J, Schlepper M. Hemodynamic and antiischemic effects of tedisamil in humans. Cardiovasc Drug Ther 1992;6:353-360.

32 Echt DS, Lee JT, Murray KT, Vorperian V, Borganelli V, Crawford DM, Roden DM. A randomized double-blind placebo-controlled dose-ranging study of intravenous UK 68798 (dofetalide) in patients with inducible sustained ventricular tachyarrhythmias. Circulation 1991;84 (4 suppl)11-714.

33 Bril A, Faivre JF, Landais L, et al. Effect of BRL-32872, a new antiarrhythmic agent, on the susceptibility to experimentally-induced triggered arrhythmias. FASEB 1994;8 (4):Abs 455.

34 What is a cardioprotective drug? Chp 1, pp2-8 in Preventing coronary artery disease. Kendall MJ, Horton RC (Eds). Martin Dunitz, London 1994.

35 Gross GJ, Auchampach JA, Maruyama M, Warltier DC, Pieper GM. Cardioprotective effects of nicorandil. J Cardiovasc Pharmacol 1992;20 (suppl 3):S22-S28.

36 Auchampach JA, Maruyama M, Cavero I, Gross GJ. The new K+ Channel opener aprikalim (RP 52891) reduces experimental infarct size in dogs in the absence of hemodynamic changes. J Pharmacol Exp Ther 1991;259:961-7.

37 Auchampach JA, Gross GJ. Reduction in myocardial infarct size by the new potassium channel opener bimakalim. J Cardiovasc Pharmacol 1994;23:554-561.

38 Cole WC, McPherson CD, Sontag D. ATP-regulated K+ channels protect the myocardium against ischemia/reperfusion damage. Circulaton Res 1991;69:571-581.

39 Purcell H, Fox K. Potassium channel activators in the management of ischaemic heart disease: a focus on nicorandil. Br J Clin Prac 1993;47:150-154.

40 Purcell H, Patel D, Mulcahy D, Fox K. Nicorandil. in Cardiovascular Drug Therapy. 2nd edition. Messerli F. WB Saunders Co, Philadelphia. 1995 (in press).

41 Gross GJ, Auchampach A, Maruyama M, Warltier DC, Pieper GM. Cardioprotective effects of nicorandil. J Cardiovasc Pharmacol 1992;20 (suppl 3):S22-S28.

42 Taira N. Nicorandil as a hybrid between nitrates and potassium channel activators. Am J Cardiol 1989;63:18J-24J.

43 Thadani U, Strauss W, Glasser SP et al. Evaluation of antianginal and anti-ischemic efficacy of nicorandil; results of a multicenter study. (Abstract). J Am Coll Cardiol 1994;1A.

44 Tsutamoto T, Kinoshita M, Nakae I et al. Absence of hemodynamic tolerance to nicorandil in patients with severe congestive heart failure. Am Heart J 1994;127:866-73.

45 Hongo M, Takenaka H, Uchikawa S, Nakatsuka T, Watanabe N, Sekiguchi M. Coronary microvascular response to intracoronary administration of nicorandil. Am J Cardiol 1995;75:246-250.

46 Ulvestam G, Diderholm E, Frithz G et al. Antianginal and anti-ischemic efficacy of nicorandil compared with nifedipine in patients with angina pectoris and coronary heart disease. A double-blind, randomized, multicenter study . J Cardiovasc Pharmacol 1992;20:S67-S73.

47 Roland E. Safety profile of an anti-anginal agent with potassium channel opening activity: an overview. Eur Heart J 1993;14 (suppl B):48-52.

48 Kloner RA, Yellon D. Does ischemic preconditioning occur in patients? J Am Coll Cardiol 1994;24:1133-42.

49 Lenz T, Wagner G. Potential role of potassium channel openers for treatment of cardiovascular disease. chp 177, pp 2953-2968, in Hypertension, pathophysiology, Diagnosis and Management, 2nd edition. Laragh JH, Brenner BM (Eds). Raven Press Ltd, New York, 1995.

50 Jaraki O, Strauss WE, Francis S, Loscalzo J, Stamler JS. Antiplatelet effects of a novel antianginal agent, nicorandil. J Cardiovasc Pharmacol 1994;23:24-30.

51 Sugimoto S, Iwashiro K, Monti F, Dawodu AA, Schiariti M, Puddu PE. The risk of myocardial stunning is decreased concentration-dependently by K-ATP channel activation with nicorandil before high K+ cardioplegia. Int J Cardiol 1995;48:11-25.

52 Ogawa N, Fukata Y, Kaneta S, Jinno Y, Fukushima H, Nishikori K. Comparison of KRN2391 with nicorandil and nifedipine on canine coronary blood flow:Antagonism by glibenclamide. J Cardiovasc Pharmacol 1992;20:11-17.

53 Kaneta S, Jinno Y, Miwa A, Fukushima H, Ogawa N. Effect of KRN2391 on venous return: comparison with other vasodilators. J Cardiovasc Pharmacol 1993;22:82-88.

54 Kaneta S, Jinno Y, Harada K, Fukushima H, Ogawa N. Tolerance to the increase in coronary blood flow induced by KRN2391. Arch Int Pharmacodyn Ther 1992; 318:21-35.

55 Ohta H, Jinno Y, Harada K, Ogawa N, Fukushima H, Nishikori K. Cardioprotective effects of KRN2391 and nicorandil on ischemic dysfunction in perfused rat heart. Eur J Pharmacol 1991;204:171-177.

56 Kitzen JM, McCallum JD, Harvey C, Morin M-E, Oshiro GT, Colatsky TJ. Potassium channel activators cromakalim and celikalim (WAY-120,491) fail to decrease infarct size in the anaesthetized canine. Pharmacol 1992;45:71-82.

57 Schelling P, Becker K-H, Lues I, Soei LK, Verdouw PD, Weygandt H. Cardioprotection by the K+ channel opener bimakalim in pigs under coronary artery occlusion and reperfusion. E Heart J 1992;13 (abstract suppl):400.

58 Atwal KS. Advances in the structure-activity relationships, mechanisms of action, and therapeutic utilities of ATP-sensitive potassium channel openers. Drug Devel Res 1994;33:250-262.

ACKNOWLEDGEMENTS

We are grateful to Drs N Beier, TJ Colatsky, GJ Gross, VM Miall-Allen, N Ogawa, MJ Sumner, and I Rumfitt, for their kind assistance in the preparation of this review; and to Drs G Edwards, C Jacques and Professor A Weston for their helpful advice and comments.

7

IS THERE A POTENTIAL ROLE FOR K_{ATP} OPENERS IN THE TREATMENT OF ANGINA?

LIONEL H OPIE

Heart Research Unit, University of Cape Town Medical School, Observatory 7925, Cape Town, South Africa.

INTRODUCTION

The discovery of the ATP-sensitive potassium channel (1) and the knowledge that cellular ATP is decreased in ischemia, has naturally focused attention on the possible role of the ATP-dependent potassium channel in early potassium loss. There is now considerable evidence that the opening of this channel is concerned with the early electrophysiological changes of ischemia, including shortening of the action potential duration and depolarization (2,3). Because these changes are thought to explain ST-segment changes that are diagnostic of exercise-induced angina, (4) it might be supposed that drugs acting as potassium channel openers would only exaggerate potassium loss and worsen ischemia. This point of view fails to recognize that (A) the major effects of the potassium channel openers are probably as vasodilators acting on the coronary vascular tree (5,6) and that (B) the shortening of the action potential duration has an important anti-ischemic effect, perhaps acting by local cardioplegia and reduced calcium ion entry, thereby decreasing the contractile activity of the ischemic segment and hence "resting" the ischemic myocardium (3,6). Hence the potassium channel openers have potential anti-ischemic and antianginal effects, as will be assessed in this chapter.

EFFECTS OF POTASSIUM CHANNEL MODULATION ON MYOCARDIAL ISCHEMIA

The effects on ischemia of potassium channel closers can be compared with the channel openers (Table1).

Table 1 Effects of potassium channel modulators on myocardial ischemia

	Potassium channel closing drugs	Potassium channel opening drugs
Early potassium loss	Lessen	Enhance
Shortened action potential	Widen	Shorten further
Depolarization	Lessen	Lessen
Early ventricular arrhythmias	Lessen	Enhance Low doses, no effect[6]
Late ventricular arrhythmias	Not known	Diminish
Torsades de pointes	Not known	Decrease
Reperfusion arrhythmias	Increase	Decrease
Reperfusion stunning	Increase	Decrease
Role in preconditioning	Block[24]	Promote[25]
Metabolic preservation of ischemic myocardium	Lessen	Enhance
Infarct size	No data	Decrease[24]
Ischemic arrest time	Lengthen	Shorten
Ischemic contracture	Increase	Decrease
Coronary vasodilation	Lessen	Enhance

See Opie[2] for other references.

Apart from the profibrillatory effect of high-dose potassium channel openers, the vasodilation and metabolic protection of the myocardium are attractive qualities. Also, the finding that lower doses of the potassium channel opener, bimakalim, markedly decreased infarct size in dogs without the high dose profibrillatory effect is of considerable interest. Very intriguing and challenging is the observation that the lowest dose of bimakalim reduced infarct size without shortening the action potential duration, hypothetically and possibly by reducing release of calcium from the sarcoplasmic reticulum (6). Thus, the overall evidence is that the potassium channel openers should be able to act as anti-ischemic agents, possibly without the dose-sensitive profibrillatory effects. An important reservation is that the benefits have largely been obtained with intracoronary administration, and that these agents may be much less anti-ischemic when given systemically (6).

QUALITIES OF AN IDEAL ANTIANGINAL AGENT

Desirable qualities are many (Table 2). First, and by definition, the agent must relieve anginal pain, best tested as an increase in "symptom-limited exercise duration" (7). This critical test parameter cannot be infallible, because it does not allow for variable-threshold or mixed angina (8). Such patients are often excluded from trials although they might in fact be the majority of those with angina (9).

The second important quality therefore is that the drug should also act against variable-threshold angina.

Third, the drug should improve the quality of life (10). For example, in one comparison a beta-blocker gave a better quality of life than a calcium antagonist, nifedipine.

Fourth, the drug should improve the duration of life - thus far an aim not yet achieved by any antianginal drug, not even for beta-blockers. The long-term benefits of beta-blockers in post-infarct patients do not necessarily transplant to patients with angina but without prior infarcts.

Fifth, the drug should be free of serious side-effects, or the side-effects should be acceptable in relation to the magnitude of the antianginal effect. For example, no beta-blocker is entirely free of respiratory side-effects, in the sense that even beta 1-selective agents are contraindicated in patients with asthma. Yet beta-blockers are generally effective without serious unacceptable side-effects. It is debatable whether the negative inotropic action of beta-blockers is a desirable or undesirable quality. The drug should not have potential pro-ischemic or profibrillatory effects.

Sixth, the drug should be able to suppress concurrent silent ischemia. Several studies have argued that silent ischemia, identified by ambulatory ECG monitoring, increases the risk for an adverse outcome. Yet, thus far only one study has found that drug treatment (by a beta-blocker, atenolol) has reduced clinical events at 1 year (11). Such

Table 2 Qualities of an ideal antianginal drug

Desirable quality	Nitrates	Beta-blockers	Calcium antagonists
Relief of effort angina	++	++	++
Relief of variable-threshold (mixed) angina	++	++ (atenolol tested)	++
Quality of life improved	++	++ (depends on drug)	++ (depends on drug)
Duration of life improved	?	?	??
Free of serious side-effects	++	+ or +/-	+ or +/-
Silent ischemia suppression	+	++[11]	+
Combines well with other antianginals	++	++	++ (depends on drug)
Ideal pharmacokinetics	+	++ (some)	+
Lack of tolerance	0	++	++
Relief of exercise-induced coronary constriction	++[13]	0,+[26]	++[14]
Decrease of heart rate	0	++	+ (non-DHPs)

non-DHPs = non-dihydropyridines, i.e. verapamil and diltiazem

clinical events were death, resuscitated ventricular tachycardia or fibrillation, myocardial infarction, hospitalization for unstable angina, aggravation of angina, or revascularization.

Seventh, the drug should be readily combinable with other categories of antianginals, because multiple therapy is common.

Eighth, the ideal drug should have ideal pharmacokinetics - a smooth duration of action over 24 hours and minimal or no liver metabolism so as to lessen the chances of interaction with other drugs metabolized by the liver.

Ninth, the action of the drug should be sustained and tolerance should not develop. Here the nitrates are the least ideal of the existing antianginals.

Tenth, for a vasodilator to act as an antianginal agent, it should be able to relieve exercise-induced coronary constriction occurring at the site of stenosis (12-14).
This requirement is probably crucial for the antianginal effect of vasodilators.

Eleventh, the heart rate should be reduced, a quality most readily obtained by beta-blockade and shared to some extent by the non-dihydropyridine calcium antagonists, verapamil and diltiazem.

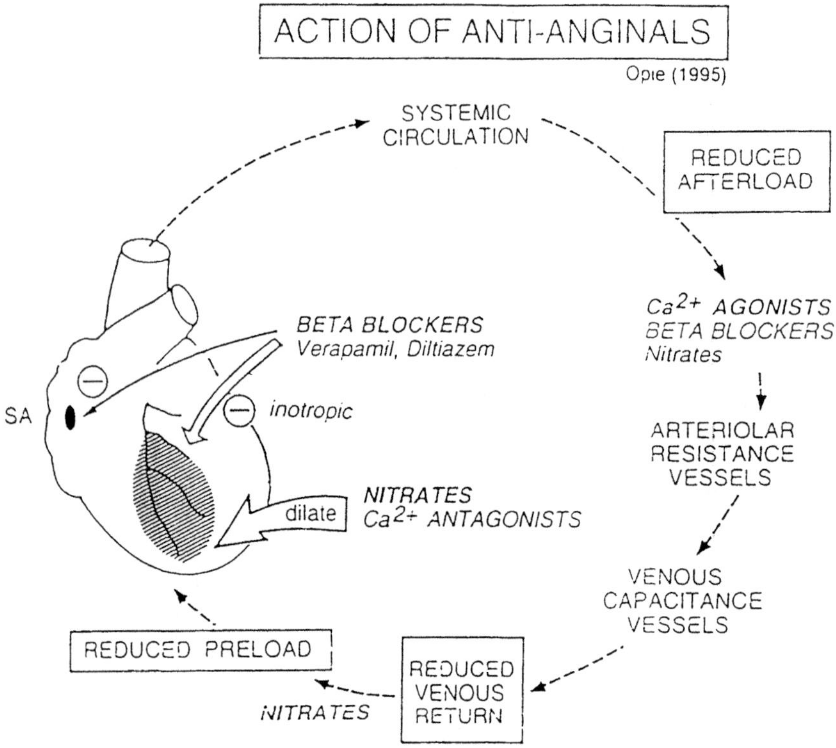

Fig 1

Major sites of action of chief existing categories of antianginal agents. SA = sinoatrial node. Fig copyright LH Opie.

Thus far, none of the major categories of existing antianginals (nitrates, beta-blockers, calcium antagonists) meet these exacting requirements. Therefore, there is indeed potential for new antianginals.

CORONARY VASODILATION

Antianginal agents in general act either via a reduction in the myocardial oxygen demand (eg. decreased heart rate and contractile activity with beta-blockers) or by vasodilation (nitrates and calcium antagonists) (Fig 1). The overall evidence is that potassium channel openers are vasodilatory at anti-ischemic doses, whereas potassium channel closers could be vasoconstrictory (Table 3). But it is not known whether or not the potassium channel openers have the crucial property of relieving exercise-induced coronary constriction.

Table 3 Effects of K^+ channel openers and blockers on coronary vascular tone

Drug	Model	Dosage	Effects
Glibenclamide[a]	Isolated rabbit heart	1 μM	Rise in coronary vascular resistance, tissue ischemia
Glibenclamide	Open chest dog, i.c.[c] infusion	55-80 μM	Vasoconstriction, metabolic ischemia
Glibenclamide	Open chest dog, i.c. infusion	50 $\mu g.kg^{-1}.min^{-1}$	Fall in coronary flow, ST-elevation
Glibenclamide + Pinacidil[b]	Open chest dog, i.c. infusion	50 $\mu g.kg^{-1}.min^{-1}$ 0/3-0.6 $\mu g.min^{-1}$	No fall in coronary flow, no ST-elevation
Glibenclamide Cromakalim[b] Pinacidil[b]	Isolated rat heart, Langendorff Isolated rat heart, Langendorff Isolated rat heart, Langendorff	1 μM 10 μM 30 μM	Increases coronary resistance Decreases coronary resistance Decreases coronary resistance
Glibenclamide	Isolated rat heart	1 or 10 μM	Coronary flow falls
Glibenclamide	Open chest dog i.v.[d]	10 $mg.kg^{-1}$	Coronary flow falls
Glibenclamide	Isolated guinea-pig heart	2 μM	Inhibits hypoxic or adenosine vasodilation
Cromakalim	Isolated guinea-pig heart	100 or 500 nM	Vasodilation
Bimakalim	Open chest dog i.c. infusion	0.1-10 μg/min	Coronary dilation, decreased infarct size[6]

a = K^+ channel blocker; b = K^+ channel opener; c = intracoronary; d = intravenous

See Hofmann and Opie[5] for other references.

At what site do they act on the coronary vascular tree? Antianginal agents, such as the nitrates and calcium antagonists, act at least in part by vasodilation of the large epicardial coronary arteries, whereas drugs that are not antianginal, such as dipyridamole, and that dilate small resistance vessels, incur the risk of a pro-anginal effect. Hence, the vasodilation caused by cromakalim in large porcine coronary arteries (15) suggest that antianginal effects are possible. A decreased systemic vascular resistance, as found in conscious pigs after myocardial infarction (16) could also contribute to a possible antianginal effect. There is, as yet, no clinical study on the possible antianginal properties of potassium channel openers.

NICORANDIL - NOT A SIMPLE ANALOGY

Nicorandil is a mixed nitrate-potassium channel opener that is thought to have antianginal properties (Table 4; for review, see Knight 17). It is often supposed that any such antianginal effects of nicorandil support the proposal that potassium channel openers should also be antianginal. Nonetheless, these arguments are diluted by experimental findings showing that nicorandil-induced dilation of large coronary arteries is due to its nitrate-like action, whereas the vasodilatory effect on small resistance coronary arteries is related to its potassium channel opening properties (18). Thus, the nitrate-like effect could explain the antianginal properties of this drug (Table 4).

Table 4 Antianginal effects of nicorandil (N) compared with other agents in stable effort angina

Author	Trial design	Patients (n)	Test period	N dose	Other agent(s)	Results
DiSomma et al[27]	R, DBl, parallel, Pl run-in	16	6 weeks	10 mg 2x for 3 weeks then 20 mg 2x	Meto 100 mg 2x	Similar effects on anginal attacks, NG use, exercise tolerance
Doring[28]	R, SBl, Pl run-in, crossover	52	4 weeks	20 mg 2x	Iso-5-MN 20 mg 2x	Similar effects on anginal attacks and exercise time
Hughes et al[29]	R, SBl, parallel, Pl run-in	37	6 weeeks	10-20 mg 2x	At 50-100 mg 2x	Similar effects on exercise time
Kinoshita et al[30]	R, SBl, no Pl	12	Single dose	30 mg 1x	Prop 40 mg; Dilt 60-120 mg	Single dose of each increased exercise time
Meeter et al[31]	R, DBl, parallel, Pl run-in	77	6 weeks	10-20 mg 2x	Prop 40-80 mg 3x	Similar effects on exercise time at 2h; no N effect at 12h
Ulvenstam et al[32]	R, DBl, parallel, nitrate run-in	58	8 weeks	10-20 mg 2x	Nif 20 mg 2x	Similar effects on exercise time

R = randomized; DBl = double-blind; SBl = single-blind; Pl = placebo; Prop = propranolol; Dilt = diltiazem; Iso-5-MN = isosorbide-5-mononitrate; Nif = nifedipine; At = atenolol; NG = nitroglycerin; 1x = once daily; 2x = twice daily; 3x = thrice daily.

Furthermore, not all studies support the proposition that nicorandil is antianginal - an important exception is contained in a preliminary communication by Thadani et al (19) in which no benefit was found when nicorandil was compared with simultaneous double-blinded placebo administration. In most other studies, except that of Meany et al, (20) the placebo-control was given in a predrug run-in period so that a benefit of concurrent placebo administration could not be excluded (Table 5).

Table 5 Effects of nicorandil (N) on exercise performance in anginal patients

Author	Trial design	Patients (n)	Test period	N dose	Result
Camm and Maltz[33]	Single drug dose	8	Acute	20-60 mg	Dose-related increase in exercise time with risk of exercise hypotension at higher dose.
Kato et al[34]	SBl, Pl, R, crossover	29	Single dose	20 mg	Improved exercise tolerance for 6h.
Meany et al[20]	DBl, R, parallel, Pl washout	46	2 weeks	10-20 mg 2x	Improved exercise time 2-12h after dose vs concurrent placebo.
Silke et al[35]	Single dose; Swan-Ganz catheter	20	Acute	20 mg	Reduced mean BP and LV filling pressure during bicycle exercise.
Thadani et al[19]	SBl, R, parallel with concurrent Pl (DBl)	83	2 weeks	10-20 mg 2x	No effect on anginal attacks or exercise time when compared with DBl Pl.

All authors except Silke et al[35] used treadmill test.
For abbreviations, see Table 4.

Extrapolation from nicorandil to the potassium channel openers must be made cautiously especially when it is considered that (A) the potassium channel openers may be up to 250 times more powerful arterial dilators than nicorandil, (16) and (B) the effect of nicorandil on large arteries such as the aorta (21) or on the large coronary arteries (18) is almost entirely that of a nitrate-like agent. It could also be argued that the myocardial protective effects of potassium channel openers (Table 1) should not be extrapolated back to nicorandil. It also follows that potassium channel openers should be evaluated as potential antianginal agents in their own right, quite apart from any results that may have been obtained with the mixed agent, nicorandil.

SIGNIFICANCE OF STUNNING

A very consistent experimental effect of potassium channel openers has been the relief of post-ischemic stunning asdiscussed in chapter 3 by Hearse. There are two particularly important clinical applications of stunning. First, acute exercise-induced angina may precipitate wall motion abnormalities for about 30 minutes after the end of exercise (22). Second, repetitive stunning may contribute to or cause hibernation (23), a serious problem in the chronically ischemic myocardium. These are two common clinical conditions. Relief of postanginal stunning has never been the subject of any clinical drug trial, nor has the repetitive ischemia associated with the hibernating heart. *Both these important clinical conditions could, theoretically, be expected to respond to potassium channel openers. In particular, relief of postanginal left ventricular dysfunction could become a new drug indication.*

SUMMARY

Basic properties of the potassium channel openers suggest metabolic anti-ischemic protection, particularly when low doses are given by the intracoronary route. Furthermore, potassium channel openers appear to be active as coronary dilators, both of the large epicardial and the distant resistance vessels. The qualities required of an ideal antianginal agent are several and not completely met by any of the existing compounds. Experimentally, the most desirable quality pointing to the probable antianginal potency of a vasodilator is relief of exercise-induced coronary constriction. There are several important differences between potassium channel openers and nicorandil, a putative antianginal drug that has mixed nitrate and potassium channel opening properties. Therefore, the results obtained with nicorandil cannot necessarily be extrapolated to potassium channel openers, particularly because nicorandil has different properties on the large and small coronary arteries. It follows that potassium channel openers should be tested for their antianginal properties in their own right and irrespective of data already obtained with nicorandil. In particular, relief of postanginal stunning could be assessed as a possible new drug indication.

REFERENCES

1. Noma A. ATP-regulated K^+ channels in cardiac muscle. Nature 1983; 305: 147-148.

2. Opie LH. Modulation of ischemia by regulation of the ATP-sensitive potassium channel. Cardiovasc Drugs Ther 1993; 7: 507-513.

3. Gasser RNA. Klein W. Contractile failure in early myocardial ischemia: Models and mechanisms. Cardiovasc Drugs Ther 1994; 8: 813-822.

4. Kubota I. Yamaki M. Shibata T, et al. Role of ATP-sensitive K+ channel on ECG ST-segment elevation during a bout of myocardial ischemia. A study on epicardial mapping in dogs. Circulation 1993; 88 [part 1]: 1845-1851.

5. Hofmann D. Opie LH. Potassium channel blockade and acute myocardial infarction: implications for management of the non-insulin requiring diabetic patient. Editorial. Eur Heart J 1993; 14: 1585-1589.

6. Yao Z, Gross GJ. Effects of the KATP channel opener bimakalim on coronary blood flow, monophasic action potential duration, and infarct size in dogs. Circulation 1994; 89: 1769-1775.

7. Thadani U. Comments on the Food and Drug Administration (FDA) Cardiac and Renal Drugs Advisory Committee Recommended Guidelines for the Conduct of Antianginal Drug Trials. In: Ardissino D, Opie LH, Savonitto S (eds), Drug Evaluation in Angina Pectoris. Kluwer Academic Publishers, Boston. 1994. 251-253.

8. Dupuis B. European Communities' Committee for Proprietary Medicinal Products (CPMP) Working Party on Efficacy of Medicinal Products. In: Ardissino D. Opie LH, Savonitto S (eds), Drug Evaluation in Angina Pectoris. Kluwer Academic Publishers. Boston, 1994. 255-258.

9. Nadazdin A, Davies GJ. Investigation of therapeutic mechanisms of atenolol and diltiazem in patients with variable-threshold angina. Am Heart J 1994; 127: 312-317.

10. Wiklund I. Quality of life assessments in clinical trials of angina pectoris. In: Ardissino D, Opie LH, Savonitto S (eds), Drug Evaluation in Angina Pectoris. Kluwer Academic Publishers, Boston, 1994, 31-40.

11. ASIST study (The Atenolol Silent Ischemia Study) - Pepine CJ, Cohn PF, Deedwania PC, et al. for the ASIST Study Group. Effects of treatment on outcome in mildly symptomatic patients with ischemia during daily life. Circulation 1994; 90: 762-768.

12. Brown BG, Lee AB, Bolson ED, Dodge HT. Reflex constriction of significant coronary stenosis as a mechanism contributing to ischemic left ventricular dysfunction during isometric exercise. Circulation 1984; 70: 18-24.

13. Gage JE, Hess OM, Murakami T, et al. Vasoconstriction of stenotic coronary arteries during dynamic exercise in patients with classic angina pectoris: reversibility by nitroglycerin. Circulation 1986; 73: 865-876.

14. Thaulow E, Guth BD, Ross J Jr. Role of calcium channel blockers in experimental exercise-induced ischemia. Cardiovasc Drugs Ther 1987; 1: 503-512.

15. Satoh K, Mori T, Yamada H, Taira N. Nicorandil as a nitrate, and cromakalim as a potassium channel opener, dilate isolated porcine large coronary arteries in an agonist-nonselective manner. Cardiovasc Drugs Ther 1993; 7: 691-699.

16. van Woerkens LJ, Baas NRA, van der Giessen WJ, Verdouw PD. Cardiovascular effects of the novel potassium channel opener bimakalim in conscious pigs after myocardial infarction: A comparative study with nicorandil. Cardiovasc Drugs Ther 1992; 6: 409-417.

17. Knight C, Purcell H, Fox K. Potassium channel openers: Clinical applications in ischaemic heart disease - Overview of clinical efficacy of nicorandil. Cardiovasc Drugs Ther 1995, in press.

18. Nakae I, Quan L, Hashimoto K, et al. Mechanism of the vasodilatory action of nicorandil on coronary circulation in dogs. Cardiovasc Drugs Ther 1994; 8: 137-145.

19. Thadani U, Strauss W, Glasser SP, et al. Evaluation of antianginal and anti-ischemic efficacy of nicorandil: Results of a multicenter study (abstr). J Am Coll Cardiol 1994; 24: 267A.

20. Meany TB, Richardson P, Camm AJ, et al. Exercise capacity after single and twice-daily doses of nicorandil in chronic stable angina pectoris. Am J Cardiol 1989; 63: 66J-70J.

21. Kreye VAW, Lenz T, Pfrunder D, Theiss U. Pharmacological characterization of nicorandil by 86Rb efflux and isometric vasorelaxation studies in vascular smooth muscle. J Cardiovasc Pharmacol 1992; 20 (Suppl 3): S8-S12.

22. Kloner RA, Allen J, Cox TA, et al. Stunned left ventricular myocardium after exercise treadmill testing in coronary artery disease. Am J Cardiol 1991; 68: 329-334.

23. Vanoverschelde J-L, Wijns W, Depre C, et al. Mechanisms of chronic regional post-ischemic dysfunction in humans. New insights from the study of noninfarcted collateral-dependent myocardium. Circulation 1993; 87: 1513-1523.

24. Tomai F, Crea F, Gaspardone A, et al. Ischemia preconditioning during coronary angioplasty is prevented by glibenclamide, a selective ATP-sensitive K+ channel blocker. Circulation 1994; 90: 700-705.

25. Cavero I, Djellas Y, Guillon J-M. Ischemic myocardial cell protection conferred by the opening of ATP-sensitive potassium channels. Cardiovasc Drugs Ther 1995; 9 (Suppl 2): 245-255.

26. Gaglione A, Hess OM, Corin WJ, et al. Is there coronary vasoconstriction after intracoronary beta-adrenergic blockade in patients with coronary artery disease? J Am Coll Cardiol 1987; 10: 299-310.

27. Di Somma S, Liguori V, Petitto M, et al. A double-blind comparison of nicorandil and metoprolol in stable effort angina pectoris. Cardiovasc Drugs Ther 1993; 7: 119-123.

28. Doring G. Antianginal and anti-ischemic efficacy of nicorandil in comparison with isosorbide-5-mononitrate and isosorbide dinitrate: Results from two multicenter, double-blind, randomized studies with stable coronary heart disease patients. J Cardiovasc Pharmacol 1992; 20 (Suppl 3): S74-S81.

29. Hughes LO, Rose EL, Lahiri A, Raftery EB. Comparison of nicorandil and atenolol in stable angina pectoris. Am J Cardiol 1990; 66: 679-682.

30. Kinoshita M, Hashimoto K, Ohbayashi Y, et al. Comparison of antianginal activity of nicorandil, propranolol and diltiazem with reference to the antianginal mechanism. Am J Cardiol 1989; 63: 71J-74J.

31. Meeter K, Kelder JC, Tijssen JGP, et al. Efficacy of nicorandil versus propranolol in mild stable angina pectoris of effort: A long-term, double-blind, randomized study. J Cardiovasc Pharmacol 1992; 20 (Suppl 3): S59-S66.

32. Ulvenstam G, Diderholm E, Frithz G, et al. Antianginal and anti-ischemic efficacy of nicorandil compared with nifedipine in patients with angina pectoris and coronary heart disease: A double-blind, randomized, multicenter study. J Cardiovasc Pharmacol 1992; 20 (Suppl 3): S67-S73.

33. Camm AJ, Maltz MB. A controlled single-dose study of the efficacy, dose response and duration of action of nicorandil in angina pectoris. Am J Cardiol 1989; 63: 61J-65J.

34. Kato K, Asanoi H, Wakabayashi C, et al. Effect of nicorandil on exercise performance in patients with effort angina: a multicenter trial using a treadmill exercise test. J Cardiovasc Pharmacol 1987; 10 (Suppl 8): S98-S103.

35. Silke B, Verma SP, Ali MS, et al. Effects of nicorandil on left ventricular hemodynamics and volume at rest and during exercise-induced angina pectoris. Am J Cardiol 1989; 63: 49J-55J.

8

K_{ATP} CHANNEL EXPLOITATION FOR TREATING MYOCARDIAL ISCHEMIA-FUTURE DIRECTIONS

GARY J GROVER
Department of Pharmacology, Bristol-Myers Squibb Pharmaceutical Research Institute, Route 206 and Provinceline Road, Princeton, New Jersey 08543-4000, USA.

INTRODUCTION

Recent years have seen an explosion of research activity on ATP-sensitive potassium (K_{ATP}) channels, particularly in excitable tissue such as smooth muscle and heart. Their metabolic gating characteristics led early investigators to postulate a role for K_{ATP} channels in the pathogenesis of myocardial ischemia. Structurally dissimilar agents with the common property of selective K_{ATP} channel opening activity have been shown to exert direct cardioprotective effects in a variety of models of myocardial ischemia (see review in reference 1). Chemical structures of selected K_{ATP} channel openers are shown in figure 1 (chemical structures numbered). This was not an expected result given the presumed deleterious effect of enhancing a repolarizing current during myocardial ischemia. Structurally dissimilar blockers of K_{ATP} channels uniformly abolish the protective effects of K_{ATP} channel openers (1-3), an effect not seen with other classes of cardioprotective agents such as calcium antagonists, sodium channel blockers, Na^{+}/Ca^{2+} exchange inhibitors, etc. (4). While these results were of interest, this area of research remained relatively quiet until the studies of Gross and his group established a potential link between K_{ATP} channel activity and the cardioprotective effects of preconditioning (5). Presently, the concept of K_{ATP} channel opening being a cardioprotective mechanism is receiving much support, with most investigators showing cardioprotective activity, although there are some variability in results which may be explained by model differences (1).

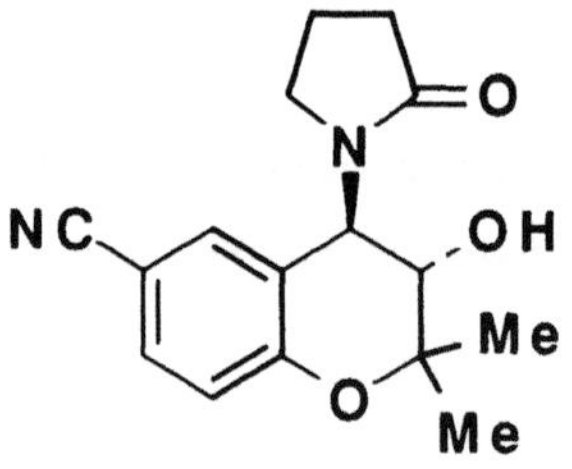

Cromakalim (**1**)

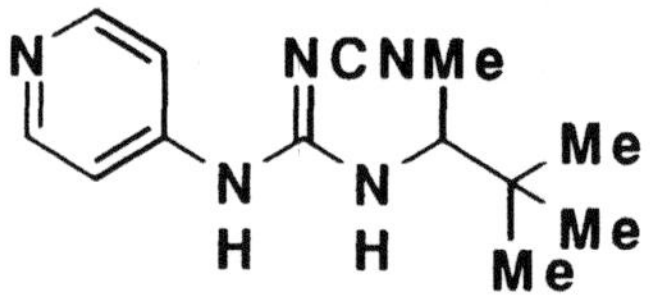

Pinacidil (**2**)

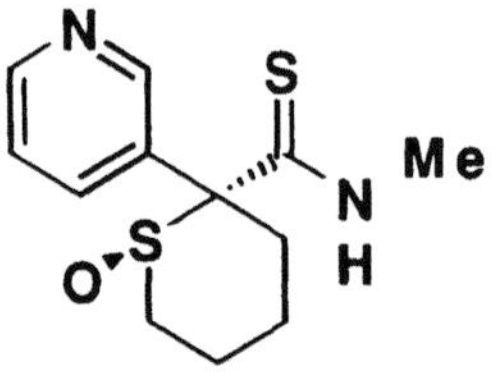

Aprikalim (**3**)

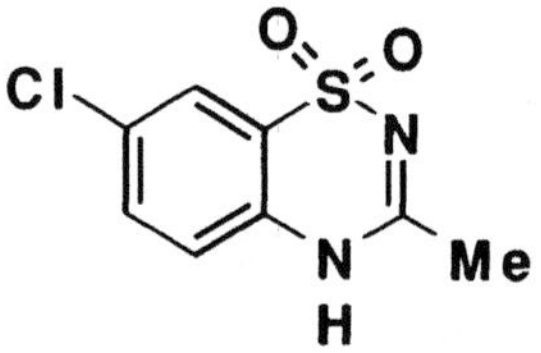

Diazoxide (**4**)

Figure 1: Chemical structures of selected K_{ATP} channel openers.

While agreement on the protective effects of K_{ATP} channels in acute myocardial ischemia is important, the next question then arises: have we maximized the activity already shown by presently existing K_{ATP} channel openers and if preconditioning is mediating by K_{ATP} channels, can this activity be reproduced or enhanced pharmacologically? The discussion of these questions forms the basis for this chapter. The first section of this chapter will focus on the current state of structure-activity (cardioprotection) relationships and how this knowledge can be used to help maximize activity and selectivity as well as develop tools for the determination of the molecular site of action for cardioprotection. Determination of the molecular site of action will then allow us to perform more rational structure-activity studies and perhaps develop more selective and potent pharmacologic agents for treating myocardial ischemia. This will enable us to develop novel chemotypes which are distinct from the currently existing K_{ATP} channel openers. Determination of the molecular site of action may also lead us to the physiologic mechanism of action, which is important for knowing which clinical indication such agents may be potentially useful for treating.

As earlier chapters in this book cover the detailed pharmacologic and physiologic data on the cardioprotective effects of currently existing K_{ATP} channel openers, I will spend no time here on this subject. I will start this chapter by discussing the current state of structure-activity determinations and how some of this work may lead to the development of novel therapeutic agents as well as tools for learning more about the molecular site of action for the cardioprotective effects of K_{ATP} channel openers. It should be pointed out that while some of the ideas discussed in this chapter have a firm experimental basis, some of the other ideas are very speculative. Any one of these speculative ideas may prove to be wrong when the proper experiments are performed.

CURRENT STATUS OF STRUCTURE ACTIVITY RELATIONSHIPS

The reference K_{ATP} channel openers originally used to determine the role of K_{ATP} channels in the pathogenesis of myocardial ischemia were not developed with myocardial ischemia in mind. Much of the early interest in these agents was in their ability to relax smooth muscle, with such indications as asthma, hypertension, and urinary incontinence being of primary interest. The early enthusiasm for the use of K_{ATP} channel openers for treating hypertension was dampened by the lack of a clear distinction from currently existing antihypertensive agents. These agents relax vascular smooth muscle in the nanomolar range (see table 1) (1,6,7). The cardioprotective potencies for nearly all K_{ATP} channel openers tested were found to be between 1-10 μM (1, see Table 1).

Table 1: Relationship of cardioprotective and vasorelaxant potencies in isolated rat hearts and methoxamine-constricted rat aorta.

	CARDIOPROTECTION (EC_{25}, μM)	VASORELAXATION (IC_{50}, μM)
BIMAKALIM	1.2	0.09
APRIKALIM (3)	2.3	0.04
LEVCROMAKALIM	2.3	0.03
PINACIDIL	1.2	0.07
BMS-180448 (15)	2.5	3.6

EC_{25} = μM for 25% increase in time to contracture

IC_{50} = μM for 50% relaxation of methoxamine constricted rat aorta

Table adapated from Grover, J Cardiovasc Pharmacol 24 (Suppl 4):S18-S27, 1994.

We have never been able to successfully treat ischemic animals systemically with standard K_{ATP} channel openers because profound hypotension usually preceded cardioprotection. Since K_{ATP} channel openers appear to predominantly dilate resistance vessels, the danger of coronary steal cannot be excluded and this has been suggested previously (8). Some investigators have been able to find protective systemic doses, although the window of efficacy is probably small (9). One of the problems with currently existing K_{ATP} channel openers (as well as most potassium channel modulators in general) is the lack of tissue selectivity (10). Thus, while currently existing K_{ATP} channel openers might be cardioprotective under the right circumstances, we did not know whether these agents were the most selective or potent cardioprotective agents. This required the determination of structure-activity relationships.

To our knowledge, no structure-activity determinations have ever been done using models of myocardial ischemia. Agents used clinically such as calcium antagonists and beta blockers were not originally designed for treatment of myocardial ischemia. These agents are certainly less than ideal as antiischemic/cardioprotective agents, most likely because of side effects such as hypotension or negative inotropic activity. Unlike agents developed for blood pressure lowering, there was no high throughput test for determining cardioprotective potency, i.e. primary screen. Another disadvantage for screening cardioprotective compounds was that only one dose or concentration of a given agent can be used per heart as ischemia is essentially an irreversible process (at least within the time frame useful for screening). Thus, we were faced with the daunting prospect of developing a primary screen which would be efficient, concentration-dependent, and predictive of *in vivo* efficacy. Since we knew that K_{ATP} channel openers were protective in isolated rat heart models of ischemia, we decided to use this test because of the relative uniformity and economical nature of the model. We also knew that the cardioprotective effects observed in this model were predictive of effects in canine models of ischemia (1). Unfortunately, many of the variables we typically measure in our rat heart model of ischemia do not respond in a clear concentration-dependent manner and are suffiently labor intensive that they do not lend themselves to rapid screening. There is one exception however and this is the time to onset of ischemic contracture during global ischemia. We found that we could construct excellent concentration-response relationships using this parameter and the concentration-response was classical in its appearance (logarithmic) (11,12). We define the time to the onset of contracture as the time during total global ischemia nesessary to observe a 5 mm Hg increase in end diastolic pressure. Using increasing concentrations of K_{ATP} channel openers, we then calculate the cardioprotective potency as an EC_{25}, defined as the concentration necessary to increase the time to contracture by 25% from vehicle-treated values (approxmately 50% of maximal response). The use of this screen has enabled us to determine detailed structure-cardioprotective activity relationships on hundreds of compounds. This test is very reliable as the results obtained can be repeated years after the first studies and the results are nearly identical. Therefore it is possible to compare cardioprotective potencies of various compounds over long periods of time.

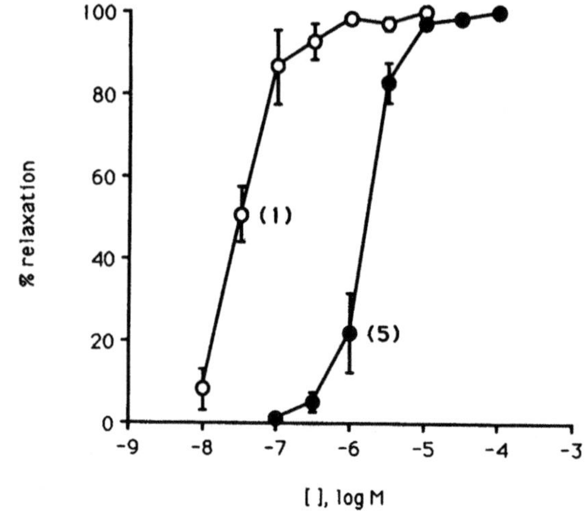

Figure 2: Concentration-response relationships of cromakalim (**1**) and phenylcyanoguanidine **5** (SQ 33,812) for relaxation of the methoxamine-contracted rat aorta. SQ 33,812 was significantly less potent as a vasodilator. Figure adapted from Atwal et al., J Med Chem 36:3971-3974, 1993.

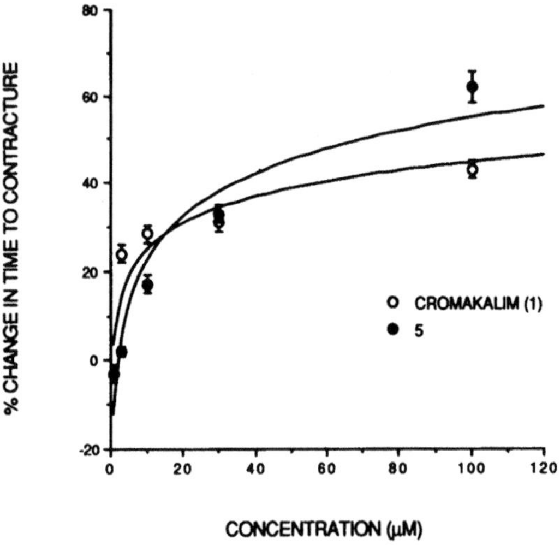

Figure 3: Concentration-response relationships for time to contracture in globally ischemic rat hearts for cromakalim (**1**) and phenylcyanoguanidine **5** (SQ 33,812). Time to contracture is defined as the time necessary during total global ischemia to increase end diastolic pressure by 5 mm Hg. Both compounds were equipotent as cardioprotective agents. Figure adapted from Atwal et al., J Med Chem 36:3971-3974, 1993.

The first question we asked was whether it was possible to separate the vasorelaxant activity from the cardioprotective activity in K_{ATP} channel openers. We chose to initially work with analogs of cromakalim, as pinacidil analogs were not as efficacious in our hands and also had other undesirable effects. We had previously screened numerous benzopyran analogs for vasodilator activity (for a hypertension program) and found numerous active and inactive compounds. We then tested these compounds for cardioprotective activity and found no correlation between vasodilator and cardioprotective activity. This separation of activities is exemplified by the phenylcyanoguanidine **5** (SQ 33,812). We explored preliminary structure-activity relationships around SQ 33,812 and these data are described in table 2 below and above in figures 2 and 3.

Table 2: Vasorelaxant and Antiischemic Potencies of Potassium Channel Openers

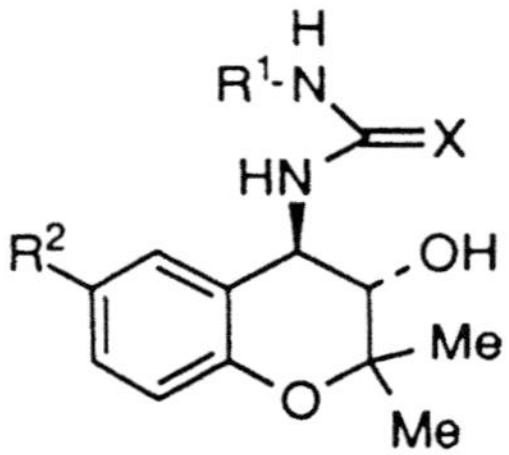

Com'd	**R1**	**R2**	**X**	**Time to Contracture[a]** EC25, μM	**Vasorelaxant potencies[b]** IC50, μM (95% C. I.)	**Ratio** EC25/IC50
5	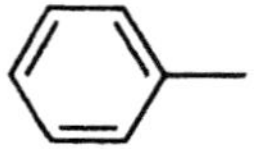	CN	NCN	11.0	1.4	7.9
6	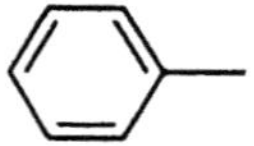	C≡CH	NCN	>30	5.4	-
7	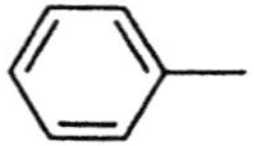	H	NCN	-[c]	72.7	-
8	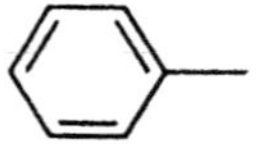	NO_2	NCN	7.2	2.0	3.6
9	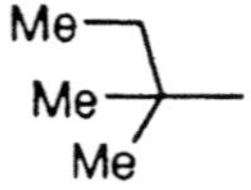	CN	NCN	20.1	29.8	0.7
10	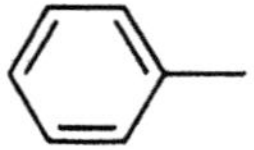	CN	O	5.1	0.8	6.4
11	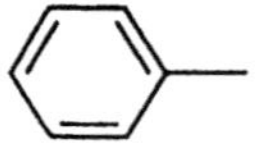	CN	S	7.7	1.7	4.5

Table 2 cont'd

12	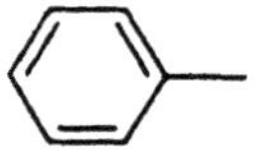	CN	NCN	6.1	1.3	4.7
13	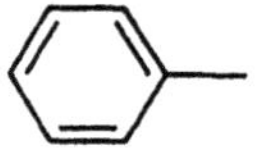	CN	NCN	>30[d]	4.2	-
14	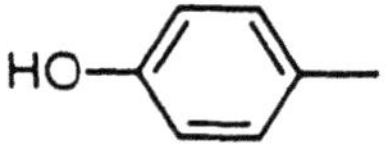	CN	NCN	33.4	2.2	15.2
15	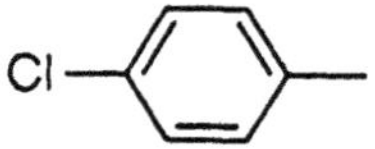	CN	NCN	2.5	1.8	1.4
16	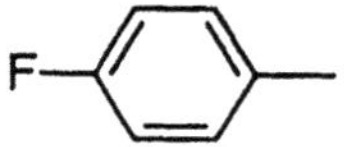	CN	NCN	3.5	1.4	2.5
17	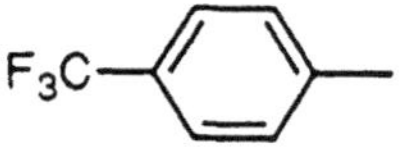	CN	NCN	13.4	8.1	1.7
1 (Cromakalim)			-	8.9	0.032	278.1

[a]Antiischemic potency was determined by measurement of EC_{25}, concentration necessary for increase in time to contracture by 25%, in the globally ischemic rat hearts. Time to contracture was defined as the time necessary during total global ischemia to increase end diastolic pressure by 5 mm Hg. Each value is an average of 3 determinations. [b]Vasorelaxant potency was assessed by measurement of IC_{50} for inhibition of methoxamine contracted rat aorta. IC_{50} is presented as a mean with 95% confidence interval in parentheses, n = 4 or higher. [c]No significant activity at 10 μM. [d]EC_{25} could not be determined due to its proischemic effects at higher than 30 μM concentrations. Table adapted from Awal et al., J Med Chem 36:3971-3974, 1993.

Despite a lack of correlation between vasodilator and cardioprotective activities, the cardioprotective activity for these compounds was always abolished by K_{ATP} channel blockers (6,12). The stereoselectivity for cardioprotective activity was assessed with the single enantiomers (3S,4R) and (3R,4S) of SQ 33,812. We found that most of the cardioprotective potency exists in the 3S,4R-enantiomer, showing stereoselectivity. Unfortunately, we found that this single enantiomer (BMS-180447) was metabolically unstable, primarily via 4-hydroxylation. Protection of this site with a 4-chloro substitution (compound **15**, BMS-180448) was found to result in a retention of the selective cardioprotective profile of BMS-180447, but had a significantly longer plasma half-life such that once a day dosing was possible.

Table 3: Comparison of the antiischemic and vasodilating potencies of cromakalim and BMS-180448

	Time to Contracture	Methoxamine Constr.	Blood Press.	Coronary Flow	
	(Rat Heart, EC_{25}, μM)[a]	Rat Aorta (IC_{50}, μM)[b]	Lowering, Dogs (ED_{20}, μmol/kg)[c]	(Rat Heart, EC_{10}, μM)[d]	Dogs (ED_{150} μmol/kg)[e]
Cromakalim	4.9	0.03	0.15	0.1	0.1
BMS-180448	2.5	3.61	21.48	4.3	>25.3

[a]EC_{25} for time to contracture is defined as the concentration necessary for a 25% increase in time to contracture.

[b]The IC_{50} is defined as the concentration necessary for relaxation by 50% of methoxamine contracted rat aorta.

[c]The ED_{20} is defined as the intravenous dose lowering mean arterial blood pressure by 20% in anesthetized dogs.

[d]The EC_{10} is defined as the concentration necessary to increase coronary flow 10% in isolated rat hearts.

[e]The ED_{150} is defined as the dose necessary for a 150% increase in coronary blood flow in dogs.

Table adapted from Grover et al. J Cardiovasc Pharmacol 25:40-50, 1995.

A detailed pharmacologic profile was determined for BMS-180448 and this was compared to cromakalim. BMS-180448 was found to be approximately 100-fold less potent as a vasorelaxant than cromakalim while having similar cardioprotective potencies (EC_{25} = 2.5 and 4.9 μM for BMS-180448 and cromakalim for increasing the time to onset of contracture, respectively) in isolated rat hearts and aortas (table 3).

The weak vasodilator as well as the cardioprotective activity were abolished by the structurally dissimilar K_{ATP} channel blockers glyburide and sodium 5-hydroxydecanoate (6,12).

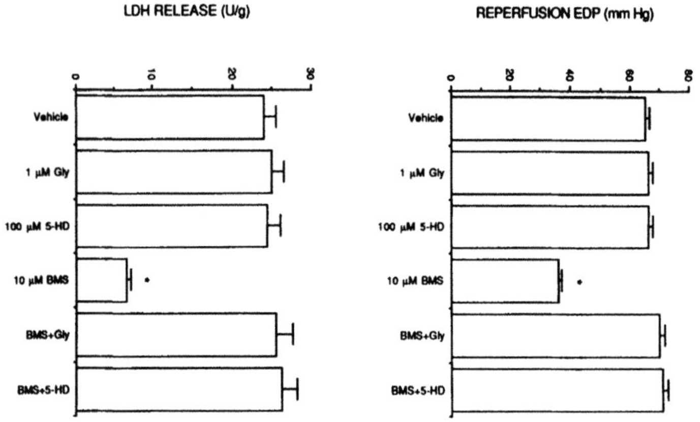

Figure 4: Effect of the K_{ATP} blockers glyburide (Gly) and 5-HD (sodium 5-hydroxydecanoate on cardioprotective effects of BMS-180448 (BMS) in isolated rat hearts subjected to 25 min global ischemia and 30 min reperfusion. BMS-180448 significantly (*$p<0.05$) reduced LDH release and end diastolic pressure (EDP). These protective effects were abolished by Gly and 5-HD. Figure adapted from Grover et al., J Cardiovasc Pharmacol 25:40-50, 1995.

As shown in figure 4, reperfusion end diastolic pressure and cumulative LDH release in ischemic/reperfused isolated rat hearts were significantly reduced by 10 μM BMS-180448 and this protective effect was completely abolished by KATP channel blockers. We also found that BMS-180448 was > 100-fold more selective for the heart relative to cromakalim in *in vivo* dog models (12) (see table 3). While most of our direct comparisons were done with cromakalim, we have found other K_{ATP} channel openers such as aprikalim, pinacidil and bimakalim to have similar profiles of activity relative to cromakalim (table 1). The only compound which we found to have nanomolar cardioprotective potency was P-1075, but this compound is also a very potent vasodilator and the ratio of cardioprotective vs vasodilator activity is similar to other reference K_{ATP} channel openers (13). We have found BMS-180448 to reduce infarct size (12) and to enhance post-ischemic recovery of contractile function after total coronary artery occlusion or after pacing-induced ischemia (14). This was done with systemic dosing, which was difficult for us to achieve with agents such as cromakalim. The dosing of BMS-180448 was calculated to be similar to the intracoronary doses of cromakalim in dogs causing significant cardioprotection (15).

The implications of these structure-activity studies are interesting and potentially important. Does this suggest receptor subtypes? Are the K_{ATP} channels that are important for mediating cardioprotection different from the K_{ATP} channels responsible for vasodilation? The selective agents described above may be useful tools to use for determining differences in binding sites. It is possible that the K_{ATP} channel responsible for cardioprotection is the same as for vasodilatation, but differences in receptor sites may exist. This would suggest that the receptors are not incorporated into the channel forming proteins, and current evidence indicates that K_{ATP} openers bind directly to K_{ATP} channels (16). Unfortunately, it is unknown if this particular binding site is relevant to cardioprotection.

We have found that it is relatively easy to increase selectivity for the heart in this series of compounds and further work has demonstrated that compounds which are virtually inactive as vasodilators are possible, while retaining glyburide-reversible cardioprotective activity. It would now be useful to increase potency for cardioprotection as the general lack of aqueous solubility of the K_{ATP} channel openers may prohibit their easy use for treating myocardial ischemia. It would therefore be useful to develop compounds with higher aqueous solubility or 100-fold increases in cardioprotective potency such that smaller amounts of drug are necessary, simplifying drug formulation. While we have learned much about synthesizing compounds which are devoid of vasorelaxant effects, one must always be aware that relatively minor changes can be made to cromakalim analogs which cause them to interact with other ion channels. For instance, the pyranoquinoline analog (BMS-188107) of cromakalim was found to block L-type calcium channels with no K_{ATP} channel activity (17). It was surprising that such a close analog of a K_{ATP} channel opener could so cleanly discriminate between different ion channels. Certainly, future development of K_{ATP} channel openers for myocardial ischemia should be done with the awareness that structural modifications of existing chemotypes could change the ion channels with which they interact.

PHYSIOLOGIC MECHANISMS OF CARDIOPROTECTION

It was initially surprising that K_{ATP} channel openers could protect ischemic myocardium, as it was thought that enhancing outward potassium current would be contraindicated during ischemia (further indicating how little we know about the mechanisms of ischemic damage). Most investigators have shown protection for K_{ATP} channel openers, and this seems to be a relatively consistent finding. Results from several laboratories suggest that such cardioprotection occurs via a direct action on the myocardium and this agrees with our findings in which vasodilator and cardioprotective activities can be dissociated in different compounds (1). This knowledge also formed the basis for our cardioprotection screen. While we know that the protective effects of K_{ATP} channels occur directly on the ischemic/reperfused myocardium, we have much to learn about their protective mechanism of action. It is important to learn the mechanism in order to develop better protective agents in the future as well as to potentially shed light on the molecular site of action of the drugs. I will therefore summarize what is known about the cardioprotective mechanism of action of

K_{ATP} channel openers and review how this information could be used for future work in the area.

An early hypothesis for the protective mechanism of action of K_{ATP} channel openers was that they would shorten action potential duration (APD) or hyperpolarize (or inhibit depolarization during ischemia) myocytes and thus inhibit the entry of calcium into the cells (18,19). This was thought to cause a cardioplegic effect, similar to that seen for calcium channel blockers. Results from several laboratories have indicated that cardioprotection can be observed at concentrations of K_{ATP} channel openers which have little effect on contractile function, distinguishing them from calcium antagonists (3,19,20). APD shortening should cause cardiodepression, if severe enough. K_{ATP} channel openers have been found to have little effect on cardiac function in normal myocardium, unlike calcium channel blockers. Interestingly, results have shown that the APD shortening activity of K_{ATP} channel openers is enhanced under ischemic conditions and thus the cardioplegic effects of K_{ATP} channel openers may only be observed during ischemia per se (21). Unpublished results from our laboratory showed that cardiac function is actually enhanced during ischemia in the presence of K_{ATP} channel openers, and thus the cardioplegic theory does not appear to be valid, at least in our model. Studies from several laboratories have also indicated that K_{ATP} channel openers can exert cardioprotective effects above that observed for cardioplegic solutions, indicating different mechanisms of action (22,23).

Despite a lack of cardiodepressant activity, K_{ATP} channel openers can protect hearts during ischemia and this effect is associated with a conservation of of the adenine nucleotide energy charge (11,24). We do not presently know if this is due to a reduced ATP hydrolysis or to enhanced synthesis. Since there is no reduction of cardiac function by K_{ATP} channel openers, a reduced ATP hydrolysis implies a more efficient utilization of energy. K_{ATP} channel openers have been shown to improve post-ischemic oxygen efficiency (25), indicating protection of the mitochondria, although it is presently unknown whether this is a primary or secondary effect of these agents. We will talk a little more about a potential mitochondrial site of cardioprotective action for K_{ATP} channel openers later in this chapter.

Yao and Gross (26) showed that it was possible to observe infarct lowering activity for bimakalim at intracoronary doses not causing monophasic APD shortening during ischemia in dogs. This would agree with the data showing a lack of correlation between cardioprotection and cardiodepression. We have recently completed a study showing that doses of dofetilide (delayed rectifier blocker, IKr) sufficient to inhibit the APD shortening effects of cromakalim before or during ischemia, did not abolish the cardioprotective effects of cromakalim (27). In the determination of our structure-activity relationships described above, we could not use APD shortening as our primary screen because of a lack of correlation between APD shortening and cardioprotection. This was unfortunate because the measurement of APD is much easier than measuring the severity of ischemia (although there are therapeutic advantages to such a separation, which will be discussed later). Nevertheless, these data suggest that the cardioprotective effects of K_{ATP} channel openers are not absolutely dependent on APD shortening. Unpublished data from our laboratories has indicated that some of the phenylcyanoguanidine analogs listed above which are relatively devoid of vasodilator activity are also devoid of APD shortening activity. Thus, it is plausible that the cardioprotective site of action is distinct from the typically described sarcolemmal K_{ATP} channel which is responsible for vasodilatation, hyperpolarization, and APD shortening (cardiac). Further structure-activity work needs to be done to determine if the agents which are weak vasodilators are also weak in terms of APD shortening and if structure-activity for this separation can be surmised.

Thus, the cardioprotective effects of glyburide-reversible agents can be dissociated, using different interventions, from their classical electrophysiologic effects. The fact that glyburide-reversible cardioprotective and electrophysiologic (as well as vasodilator) effects can be separated in different chemotypes suggests the possibility of distinct sites of action for cardioprotection and for vasodilation or APD shortening. This indicates interesting possibilities in terms of our mechanistic thinking as well as for the clinical use of these agents. It must be pointed out that the data discussed above can also suggest that the cardioprotective effects of K_{ATP} channel openers are independent of K_{ATP} channels altogether. While this is possible, it is difficult to believe that the uniform cardioprotective effects seen with structurally diverse chemotypes with the common activity of K_{ATP} channel opening is due to a "nonspecific" action which is not related to K_{ATP} channels. It is equally hard to believe that structurally diverse agents (glyburide, sodium 5-hydroxydecanoate) with the common feature of blocking K_{ATP} channels also abolish the cardioprotective effects of all K_{ATP} channel openers via a "nonspecific" effect. Therefore, I believe that the K_{ATP} channel openers are protecting the myocardium by some interaction with a K_{ATP} channel. What we do not know is the nature of this interaction. *One exciting possibility is that future development of K_{ATP} channel openers for treating myocardial ischemia can be based around enhancing cardioprotective potency while minimizing APD shortening. This would reduce the possibility of aggravating reentrant arrhythmias with this class of agents and this will be discussed in more detail later in this chapter.*

MOLECULAR SITE OF ACTION OF K_{ATP} CHANNEL OPENERS

From the preceding discussion, it becomes apparent that future developments in our understanding of the cardioprotective mechanism of K_{ATP} channel openers as well as the future development of K_{ATP} channel openers for the treatment of myocardial ischemia depend on the elucidation of the molecular site of action of these agents. This would provide a more efficient means of developing novel compounds with better and / or more selective activity. Knowledge of the relevant binding site would allow us to more rationally design agents for treating ischemia as it would be easier to model potentially new chemotypes. Unfortunately, not much progress has been made in this area.

Showing specific binding of K_{ATP} channel openers in any tissue has been difficult, although some work has been done. Specific binding for a potent cyanoguanidine, tritiated P-1075, was found by Bray and Quast in vascular smooth muscle (28). This study was performed in endothelium-denuded rat aortic rings. This binding was of high affinity (K_D = 6 nM) and was inhibited by structurally diverse K_{ATP} channel openers, suggesting a common binding site. This binding site was not only recognized by the various classes of K_{ATP} channel openers, but the binding was correlated to physiologic activity (Rb^+ efflux) in smooth muscle. Interestingly, the glyburide site in their model appears to be coupled in a negative allosteric manner to the binding site for the K_{ATP} channel openers. The pharmacologic data, unfortunately, suggests that this K_{ATP} channel binding site may not be relevant for cardioprotection (although this is far from a proven fact). Similar studies have not been done in the heart and it would be interesting to determine if specific binding can be found. The cardiac selective agents such as BMS-180448 or its congeners cited above might be useful tools for dissecting the relevant cardioprotective site of action as they appear to be devoid of the classical effects of other K_{ATP} channel openers. If specific binding for these selective agents could be found, then it will be possible to determine the protein binding site, and thus learn the potential molecular site of action. For a review on the pharmacologic data pertaining to potential K_{ATP} channel modulator binding sites, see reference 29.

A rat heart K_{ATP} channel has been cloned and heterologously expressed in human and hamster kidney epithelial cell lines (16). Single channel studies indicated that application of 1 mM Mg-ATP (inside-out patches) inhibited channel activity, and this was reversed by washout. The cloned channels showed rundown in a manner which was similar to native channels. The single channel conductance, rectification and kinetics of this cloned K_{ATP} channel were similar to those for native channels. These cloned channels were found to be activated by pinacidil, but were not inhibited by glyburide, suggesting that the channel and glyburide binding sites are distinct. It is presently unknown if this K_{ATP} channel represents the relevant cardioprotective site of action, but it would certainly be interesting to determine if the pyranyl cyanoguanidines such as BMS-180448 would bind or interact with this channel.

Pharmacologic data suggests that the relevant cardioprotective site may be different from the classical K_{ATP} channel opener site. It would be of interest to determine if this is true and if another K_{ATP} channel is involved. One interesting (and very speculative) place to search for such a binding site may be the mitochondria. A potassium channel which is inhibited by ATP and glyburide has been found in mitochondria from rat liver (30). Paucek et al. (31,32) also showed the existence of a mitochondrial K_{ATP} channel in beef heart and rat liver. In these studies, they reported the reconsititution and purification of an inner membrane K_{ATP} channel. This mitochondrial K_{ATP} channel has electrophysiologic properties that are similar to the channels found on the plasmalemma. In a further extension of their work on mitochondrial K_{ATP} channels, Paucek et al. (31) showed that cromakalim and several cromakalim analogs opened this mitochondrial K_{ATP} channel at 1 μM. This is remarkably similar to the cardioprotective concentrations found for these agents. One means of determining if this is the cardioprotective site of action would be to take agents such as BMS-180448 which are devoid of classical sarcolemmal K_{ATP} channel opening activity and determine if they are binding selectively to a mitochondrial site. In theory, BMS-180448 should not bind to the sarcolemmal K_{ATP} channel while binding to the mitochondrial site. Garlid's laboratory is now attempting to elucidate the amino acid sequence of a 54 kDa protein which predominates in the purified fraction, although this does not guarantee that this is the relevant protein. The identification of such a binding site would spur novel drug development to selectively bind and activate this receptor with high potency. It would also be possible to move away from the currently existing K_{ATP} channel opener chemotypes.

If mitochondrial K_{ATP} channels are involved in the cardioprotective effects of K_{ATP} channel openers, then it would be useful, as well as interesting, to detemine the mechani for this protection. It is unknown how the mitochondrial K_{ATP} channel could be or physiologically given the high affinity for ATP, but Paucek et al. (32) speculate that an unknown endogenous activator reduces ATP affinity. These same investigators suggest several possible physiologic roles for mitochondrial K_{ATP} channels. Mitochondrial K_{ATP} channels may open under appropriate conditions to expand matrix volume associated with protein synthesis and expansion of membranes. They also speculate on an energy dissipating role for this channel such that during episodes of low demand of energy, this would provide a mechanism for heat production for the cell. At the present time it is difficult to understand how these functions could participate in cardioprotection.

CLINICAL INDICATIONS FOR CARDIOPROTECTIVE K_{ATP} CHANNEL OPENERS: PRESENT AND FUTURE

Much excitement has been generated by the findings, in both animals,and especially in man, that K_{ATP} channels may be involved in the mechanism of preconditioning. These data strongly indicate that appropriately designed K_{ATP} channel openers may mimic an endogenous cardioprotective mechanism. This has generated much interest in the possibility that K_{ATP} channel openers may have a potential therapeutic role in acute myocardial ischemia.

Currently, most experimental data suggest that K_{ATP} channel openers will be efficacious for treatment of acute myocardial infarction. Given the nature these agents, they will have to be given early into an ischemic event. It is also possible that K_{ATP} channel openers can attenuate mortality in subsequent ischemic episodes. Unfortunately, little data exists on the efficacy of K_{ATP} openers in models of chronic stable angina, which is an important indication, both because of the size of the patient population as well as the relative ease of clinical testing. Results from my laboratory showed that K_{ATP} channel openers have little effect on ST-segment shifts during pacing-induced ischemia, but do enhance post-pacing induced ischemic contractile function (33). Nicorandil has been found to be efficacious in treating stable angina, although the interpretation of these data are difficult because of the nitrate-like activity of this compound. Certainly, most clinical investigators will initially test their respective K_{ATP} channel openers in chronic stable angina patients and it will remain to be seen whether or not more selective (in terms of K_{ATP} channel opening as well as tissue) agents are efficacious. If they are not, the difficult decision will have to be reached as to whether to pursue more severe ischemic indications such as unstable angina or infarction, which are costly and time consuming studies. It is currently unknown whether currently available K_{ATP} channel openers have a sufficient therapeutic window because of hypotension and as such more selective and/or potent K_{ATP} channel openers need to be developed.

One indication that could be relatively easy to test for is the use of K_{ATP} channel openers as adjunctive therapy to cardioplegia in surgical patients. While this population of patients is smaller than that for stable angina, the end points for protection are fairly clear. It has also been shown experimentally that K_{ATP} channel openers can exert additional protective effects over that conferred by depolarizing cardioplegic solutions (22,23).

The use of K_{ATP} channel openers for treating coronary artery disease patients (both for clinical trials as well as treatment) will also raise the question of co-treatment with sulfonylureas. First, clinicals trials must use sulfonylurea treatment as an exclusion criteria. Secondly, patients with type II diabetes who are treated with sulfonylureas will most likely not expect to get a cardioprotective effect of K_{ATP} channel openers. Since diabetics are greatly at risk for cardiac events and since a high number of patients are treated with sulfonylureas, this becomes an important question. Of course there are alternatives to sulfonylureas such as biguanide antidiabetic agents and these agents need to be tested for K_{ATP} channel blocking activity (34). It may also be possible to develop sulfonylureas with little activity in cardiac tissue. The use of such agents will be relevant because of the possibility that sulfonylureas such as glyburide can abolish preconditioning in man (35).

K_{ATP} channels exist in several tissue types including kidney, brain, and skeletal muscle (36-39). K_{ATP} channels exist in certain parts of the brain (e.g. hippocampus) where they may modulate the release of excitatory amino acids by inhibiting calcium entry into synaptic terminals via hyperpolarization (40). K_{ATP} channel openers, may therefore be useful in the treatment of cerebral ischemia. Unfortunately, most K_{ATP} channel openers do not readily cross the blood-brain barrier. Future drug development could be focused on developing K_{ATP} openers which cross the blood-brain barrier and could be potentially used for both myocardial and cerebral ischemia. This is a classical medicinal chemistry question and structure-activity studies should readily yield agents which can cross the blood-brain barrier. Skeletal muscle is also richly invested with K_{ATP} channels (36). It is also presently uniknown if K_{ATP} openers can protect ischemic skeletal muscle. Some experimental evidence indicates that non-tissue selective K_{ATP} openers can have beneficial effects on skeletal muscle ischemia, although it is presently unknown if this is due to a hemodynamc effect or due to a direct effect on the skeletal muscle (41). There is little in the way of efficacious pharmacologic therapy for peripheral vascular disease. Vasodilators have been uniformly disappointing for treatment of this disease, possibly due to a lack of selectivity or due to a lack of flow reserve in this tissue. A direct protective effect on ischemic skeletal muscle would be a novel approach to a clinically important disease which has consistently defied any efforts to achieve effective pharmacotherapy.

K_{ATP} channel openers have been hypothesized to aggravate arrhythmias, particulary of the reentrant type, although not all studies have shown this to be true (42, review 43-also see chapter by Janse & Wilde). The finding that the cardioprotective effects of K_{ATP} channel openers can be separated from APD shortening is potentially important. Even more important, compounds can be synthesized which retain glyburide-reversible cardioprotective effects while being nearly devoid of APD shortening activity. This not only suggests the possibility of a lowered propensity for increasing arrhythmias, but suggests that such agents could be safely used in combination with Class III antiarrhythmic agents. Because of a lack of APD shortening effects, these K_{ATP} channel openers would not be expected to attenuate the APD lengthening effects of Class III agents and thus these agents would not lose their anti-arrhythmic or antifibrillatory activity.

SUMMARY

There is currently much interest in the involvement of K_{ATP} channels in myocardial ischemia. It is presently unknown how K_{ATP} channel openers will fit in as a therapeutic tool. Certainly most investigators agree that K_{ATP} channel openers are protective. The important issues which need to be addressed are whether currently existing agents are optimal for treating acute myocardial ischemia. Work must continue to determine the physiological as well as molecular mechanism of action for cardioprotection with K_{ATP} channel openers. Discovery of the molecular binding site may markedly increase our understanding of how these agents work and thus increase our ability to optimize cardioprotective activity.

REFERENCES

1. Grover GJ, 1994, Protective effects of ATP-sensitive potassium-channel openers in experimental myocardial ischemia. J Cardiovasc Pharmacol 24 (Suppl. 4):S18-S27.

2. Auchampach JA, Maruyama M, Cavero I, Gross GJ, 1991, The new K^+ channel opener aprikalim (RP 52891) reduces experimental infarct size in dogs in the absence of hemodynamic changes. J Pharmacol Exp Ther 259:961-967.

3. Ohta H, Jinno Y, Harada K, Ogawa N, Fukushima, Nishikore J, 1991, Cardioprotective effects of KRN2391 and nicorandil on ischemic dysfunction in perfused rat heart. Eur J Pharmacol 204:171-177.

4. Sargent CA, Smith MA, Dzwonczyk S, Sleph PG, Grover GJ, 1991, Effect of potassium channel blockade on the anti-ischemic actions of mechanistically diverse agents. J Pharmacol Exp Ther 259:97-103.

5. Gross GJ, Auchampach JA, 1992, Blockade of ATP-sensitive potassium channels prevents myocardial preconditioning in dogs. Circ Res 70:223-233.

6. Atwal KS, Grover GJ, Ahmed S, Ferrara FN, Harper TW, Kim KS, Sleph PG, Dzwonczyk S, Russell AD, Moreland S, McCullough JR, Normandin DE, 1993, Cardioselective anti-ischemic ATP-sensitive potassium channel openers. J Med Chem 36:3971-3974.

7. Quast U, Cook NS, 1989, Moving together: K^+ channel openers and ATP-senstivie K^+ channels. Trends Pharmacol 10:431-435.

8. Sakamoto S, Liang C, Stone CK, Hood WB, 1989, Effects of pinacidil on myocardial blood flow and infarct size after acute left anterior descending coronary artery occlusion and reperfusion in awake dogs with and without a coexisting left circumflex coronary artery stenosis. J Cardiovasc Pharmacol 14:747-755.

9. Auchampach JA, Maruyama M, Cavero I, Gross G, 1992, Pharmacologic evidence for a role of ATP-dependent potassium channels in myocardial stunning. J Pharmacol Exp Ther 86:311-319.

10. Atwal KS, 1992, Modulation of potassium channels by organic molecules. Med Res Rev 12:569-591.

11. Grover GJ, Newburger J, Sleph PG, Dzwonczyk S, Taylor SC, Ahmed SZ, Atwal KS, 1991. Cardioprotective effects of the potassium channel opener cromakalim: Stereoselectivity and effects on myocardial adenine nucleotides. J Pharmacol Exp Ther 257:156-162.

12. Grover GJ, McCullough JR, D'Alonzo AJ, Sargent CA, Atwal KS, 1995, Cardioprotective profile of the cardiac-sensitive potassium channel opener BMS-180448. J Cardiovasc Pharmacol 25:40-50.

13. Sargent CA, Sleph PG, Dzwonczyk S, Normandin D, Antonaccio MJ, Grover GJ, 1993, Cardioprotective effects of the cyanoguanidine potassium channel opener P-1075. J Cardiovasc Pharmacol 22:564-570.

14. Grover GJ, Parham CS, 1994, Protective effects of the cardioselective ATP-sensitive potassium channel opener BMS-180448 in two stunned myocardium models. J Am Coll Cardiol 23:42A.

15. Grover GJ, Dzwonczyk S, Parham CS, Sleph PG, 1990, The protective effects of cromaklim and pinacidil on reperfusion function and infarct size in isolated perfused rat hearts and anesthetized dogs. Cardiovasc Drugs Ther 4:465-474.

16. Ashford MLJ, Bond CT, Blair TA, Adelman JP, 1994, Cloning and functional expression of a rat heart K_{ATP} channel. Nature 370:456-459.

17. Grover GJ, Sleph PG, Dzwonczyk S, McCullough JR, 1993, Cardioprotective effects of a novel calcium antagonist related to the structure of cromakalim. J Pharmacol Exp Ther 267:102-107.

18. Auchampach JA, Maruyama M, Gross GJ, 1994, Cardioprotective actions of potassium channel openers. Eur Heart J 15 (Suppl C0 15:89-94.

19. Grover GJ, McCullough JR, Sleph PG, Conder ML, Henry D, 1989, Protective effects of potassium channel activation in myocardial ischemia: Beneficial action of pinacidil and BRL 34915 (cromakalim) and reversal with glyburide. J Pharmacol Exp Ther 251: 98-104.

20. Galiñanes M, Shattock MJ, Hearse DJ, 1992, Effects of potassium channel modulation during global ischaemia in isolated rat heart with and without cardioplegia. Cardiovasc Res 26:1063-1068.

21. Cole WC, McPherson CD, Sontag D, 1991, ATP-regulated channels protect the myocardium against ischemia/reperfusion damage. Circ Res 69:571-581.

22. Hosoda H, Sunamori M, Watanabe M, Suzuki A, 1992, Effect of pinacidil combined with potassium cardioplegia on myocardial viability in hypothermic global ischemia follwed by reperfusion.
J Mol Cell Cardiol 24 (Suppl 1):S76 (Abstr).

23. Pignac J, Bourgouin J, Dumont L, 1993, Cold cardioplegia and the K^+ channel modulator aprkalim: Improved cardioprotection in isolated ischemic rabbit hearts. Can J Physiol Pharmacol 72:126-132.

24. McPherson CD, Pierce GN, Cole WC, 1993, Ischemic cardioprotection by ATP-sensitive potassium channels involves high-energy phosphate preservation. Am J Physiol 265:H1809-H1818.

25. Grover GJ, Sleph PG, Dzwonczyk S, 1990, Pharmacologic profile of cromakalim in the treatment of myocardial ischemia in isolated rat hearts and anesthetized dogs. J Cardiovasc Pharmacol 16:853-864.

26. Yao Z, Gross GJ, 1994, Effects of the K_{ATP} opener bimakalim on coronary blood flow, monophasic action potential duration, and infarct size in dogs. Circulation 89:1769-1775.

27. Grover GJ, D'Alonzo AJ, Parham CS, Darbenzio RB, 1995, Cardioprotection with the K_{ATP} opener cromakalim is not corrleated with ischemic myocardial action potential shortening. J Cardiovasc Pharmacol (In Press).

28. Bray KM, Quast U, 1992, A specific binding site for K^+ channel openers in rat aorta. J Biol Chem 267:11689-11692.

29. Edwards G, Weston AH, 1993, The pharmacology of ATP-sensitive potassium channels. Ann Rev Pharmacol Toxicol 33:597-637.

30. Inoue I, Nagase H, Kishi K, Higuti T, 1991, ATP-sensitive K^+ channel in the mitochondrial inner membrane. Nature 352:244-7.

31. Paucek P, Yarov-Yarovoy V, Sun X, Garlid KD, 1995, Physiological and pharmacological activators of the mitochondrial KATP channel. Biophys J 68:A145 (Abstract).

32. Paucek P, Mironova G, Mahdi F, Beavis AD, Woldegiorgis G, Garlid KD, 1992, Reconstitution and partial purification of the glibenclamide-sensitive, ATP-dependent K^+ channel from rat liver and beef heart mitochondria. J Biol Chem 36:26062-26069.

33. Grover GJ, Parham CS, 1994, Protective effects of the cardioselective ATP-sensitive potassium channel opener BMS-180448 in two stunned myocardium models. J Am Coll Cardiol 23:42A (Abstract).

34. Marchetti P, Navalesi R, 1989, Pharmacokinetic-pharmacodynamic relationships of oral hypoglycaemic agents: An update. Clin Pharmacokin 16:100-128.

35. Tomai F, Crea F, Gaspardone A, Versaci G, De Paulis R, Penta de Peppo A, Chiariello L, Gioffre PA, 1994, Ischemic preconditioning during coronary angioplasy is prevented by glibenclamide, a selective ATP-sensitive K^+ channel blocker. Circulation 90:700-705.

36. Spruce AE, Standen NB, Stanfield PR, 1985, Voltage-dependent ATP-sensitive potassium channels of skeletal muscle membrane. Nature 316:736-738.

37. Grigg JJ, Anderson EG, 1989, Glucose and sulfonylureas modify different phases of the membrane potential change during hypoxia in rat hippocampal slices. Brain Res 489:302-310.

38. Treherne JM, Ashford MLJ. The regional distribution of sulfphonylurea binding sites in rat brain. Neuroscience 1991;40:523-31.

39. Wang W, White S, Geibel J, Giebisch G, 1990, A potassium channel in the apical membrane of rabbit thick ascending limb of Henle's loop. Am J Physiol 258:F244-F253.

40. Heurteaux C, Bertaina V, Widman C, Lazdunski M, 1993, K^+ channel openers prevent global ischemia-induced expression of *c-fos*, *c-jun*, heat shck proten, and amyloid beta-protein precursor gens and neuronal death in rat hippocampus. Proc Natl Acad Sci USA 90:9431-9435.

41. Angersbach D, Nicholson CD, 1988, Enhancement of muscle blood cell flux and pO2 by cromakalim and other compounds enhancing membrane K^+ conductance, but not by Ca^{2+} antagonists or hydralazine, in an animal modle of occlusive artertial disease. Naunyn-Schmiedeberg's Arch Pharmacol 337:341-346.

42. Chi L, Uprichard ACG, Lucchesi BR, 1990, Profibrillatory actions of pinacidil in a conscious canine model of sudden coronary death. J Cardiovasc Pharmacol 15:452-462.

43. D'Alonzo AJ, Grover GJ, 1994, Potassium channel openers are unlikely to be proarrhythmic in the diseased human heart. Cardiovasc Res 28:924-925.

INDEX

Note: Page numbers in italics refer to figures; page numbers followed by *t* indicate tables.